The Effectiveness of Health Impact Assessment

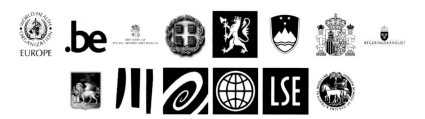

EUROPE

The European Observatory on Health Systems and Policies supports and promotes evidence-based health policy-making through comprehensive and rigorous analysis of health systems in Europe. It brings together a wide range of policy-makers, academics and practitioners to analyse trends in health reform, drawing on experience from across Europe to illuminate policy issues.

The European Observatory on Health Systems and Policies is a partnership between the World Health Organization Regional Office for Europe, the Governments of Belgium, Finland, Greece, Norway, Slovenia, Spain and Sweden, the Veneto Region of Italy, the European Investment Bank, the Open Society Institute, the World Bank, the London School of Economics and Political Science and the London School of Hygiene & Tropical Medicine.

The Effectiveness of Health Impact Assessment

Scope and limitations of supporting decision-making in Europe

Edited by

Matthias Wismar

Julia Blau

Kelly Ernst

Josep Figueras

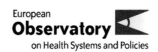

Keywords:
HEALTH STATUS INDICATORS
RISK ASSESSMENT
EVIDENCE-BASED MEDICINE
SOCIOECONOMIC FACTORS
PROGRAM EVALUATION
DECISION MAKING
POLICY MAKING
PUBLIC HEALTH ADMINISTRATION
CASE REPORTS
EUROPE

Please address requests about the publication to: Publications, WHO Regional Office for Europe, Scherfigsvej 8, DK-2100 Copenhagen Ø, Denmark

Alternatively, complete an online request form for documentation, health information, or for permission to quote or translate, on the Regional Office web site (http://www.euro.who.int/PubRequest)

ISBN 978 92 890 7295 3 (print)
ISBN 978 92 890 7296 0 (ebook)

Printed in the United Kingdom by The Cromwell Press, Trowbridge, Wilts.

Contents

Part III: The Effectiveness of Health Impact Assessment: Case Studies

Part IV: The Effectiveness of Integrating Health in Other Impact Assessments: Case Studies

List of tables, figures and boxes

The abbreviation CS refers to those tables, figures and boxes within the case studies sections.

Part III

Foreword

Making decisions at any level requires judgement, and judgement must be based on the best available knowledge and information about all the consequences of the action to be taken. Many decisions made in a wide range of policy areas have an impact on health – sometimes to a surprising degree. How many developers of new roads, for example, take into account the true impacts of those roads on health? A new bypass road may solve traffic congestion problems, but the additional pollution and noise, and discouragement from walking or cycling along that route might well have an adverse effect on the health of the population in the area.

All governments will seek to avoid these kinds of problems resulting from decision-making. However, gathering the necessary information to support a good decision is not an easy task. Tools such as health impact assessment (HIA) can make a real difference in enabling policy-makers to predict the consequences of proposals. As the mapping exercise and case studies in this volume demonstrate, HIA can be used across all sectors and at all levels of decision-making.

Impact assessment is already regularly undertaken at European level. The European Commission (EC) has made it a priority to carry out impact assessments which capture social, economic and environmental impacts on all major new proposals. Impacts on health and health systems are considered as part of this comprehensive procedure. Further to this, the EC is working with European Union (EU) Member States to develop methodologies and tools for addressing health and health systems in decision-making, in particular through the High Level Group on Health Services and Medical Care.

Given the considerable social, political and economic diversity between the EU Member States, HIA needs to be flexible enough to adapt to each specific purpose and context. It is evident, however, that a common thread runs through HIAs in whichever situation they are used. This makes the exchange of experiences and evidence indispensable. As part of the project "Effectiveness of Health Impact Assessment", supported by EC funding, the European Observatory on Health Systems and Policies has used its expert networks to bring together valuable evidence of this type. Case studies from a multitude of countries are combined in one volume, to show the reality of HIA use across Europe.

When implementing HIA, or integrating health into other forms of impact assessment, we can learn from the experiences of all these countries, regardless of the sector they involve or the level at which they are carried out.

I welcome this book as a valuable resource for all those working with HIA.

Robert Madelin
Director General for Health and Consumer Protection
European Commission

August 2007

Acknowledgements

We are grateful for the generous contributions made to this project by numerous individuals and organizations, and in particular the 21 partners of the "Effectiveness of Health Impact Assessment" (HIA) project. We are heavily indebted to our chapter authors, whose commitment of both time and knowledge made this study possible.

We are most thankful to the members of our project's steering committee: Caroline Costongs (EuroHealthNet, Belgium), Eva Elliott (Cardiff University, United Kingdom), Gabriel Gulis (University of Southern Denmark), Alison Golby (Cardiff University, United Kingdom), Loes van Herten (TNO Quality of Life, the Netherlands), Kerttu Perttilä (STAKES, Finland), Timo Ståhl (STAKES, Finland) and Ingrid Stegeman (EuroHealthNet, Belgium). Their commitment in supporting the project by reviewing the progress of project tasks and specifically the development of the conceptual frameworks and methodologies was invaluable.

We are also deeply indebted to the external experts, and would like to thank Ceri Breeze (National Assembly for Wales), Clémence Dallaire (Université Laval, Canada), Arne Marius Fosse (Directorate for Health and Social Affairs, Norway), France Gagnon (University of Ottawa, Canada), John Kemm (West Midlands Public Health Observatory, United Kingdom), Marco Martuzzi (WHO Regional Office for Europe) and Matthew Soeberg (WHO Regional Office for Europe).

Louise Nilunger (Karolinska Institute, Sweden) and Jane Parry (University of Birmingham, United Kingdom) reviewed the questionnaire for the mapping exercise while Marco Martuzzi conducted a pre test. Tony van Loon (Vrije Universiteit Brussel, Belgium) provided guidance for the development of methodologies for the effectiveness analysis, in particular the interview questions and the user guide. Alison Golby conducted a pre test using the resource package for the interviews.

Ben Cave (Ben Cave Associates, United Kingdom) and Louise Nilunger acted as external reviewers for the draft case studies. We benefited greatly from their helpful comments and suggestions.

We would like to thank our Swedish project partner, the National Institute for Public Health and the Wales Centre for Health for hosting project meetings in 2005 and 2006 respectively.

We would also like to thank the participants of our workshops for their valuable comments on the preliminary results. Workshops were conducted during the International Union for Health Promotion and Education (IUHPE) 2005 conference in Stockholm, the annual German health promotion conference (DGSMP) 2005, the 7th International HIA conference in Cardiff 2006 and the European Public Health Association (EUPHA) conference 2006 in Montreux. We would also like to thank the organizers of the HIA conference in Turin in 2006.

We are also grateful that the Health Systems Working Party has provided us with the opportunity to present the preliminary results of this study for discussion with European project leaders.

Many thanks to the European Observatory on Health Systems and Policies team in Brussels, and to Renee Lertzman for her editorial support. This book would not have been possible without the hard work throughout the project of the publication team, in particular Giovanna Ceroni, Jonathan North, Nicole Satterley and Caroline White.

This project was co-funded by the European Commission, under the Public Health Programme. We would like to thank our technical and financial focal points in the European Commission for their great support.

Contributors

Contributors to Chapters 1–4:

Franz Baro (*WHO Collaborating Centre on Health and Psychosocial Factors, Belgium*), Julia Blau (*European Observatory on Health Systems and Policies, Belgium*), Mojca Gabrijelčič Blenkuš (*Institute of Public Health of the Republic of Slovenia*), Konrade von Bremen (*Institute of Health Economics and Management (IEMS), University of Lausanne*), Eva Elliott (*Cardiff Institute of Society, Health and Ethics, Cardiff University School of Social Sciences*), Kelly Ernst (*European Observatory on Health Systems and Policies, Brussels*), Rainer Fehr (*Institute of Public Health (LÖGD), Germany*), Alison Golby (*Cardiff Institute of Society, Health and Ethics, Cardiff University School of Social Sciences*), Gabriel Gulis (*University of Southern Denmark, Unit of health promotion research, Esbjerg*), Loes van Herten (*Netherlands Organisation for Applied Scientific Research (TNO)*), Tapani Kauppinen (*National Research and Development Centre for Welfare and Health (STAKES), Finland*), John Kemm (*West Midlands Public Health Observatory, Birmingham*), Teresa Lavin (*Institute of Public Health in Ireland*), Odile Mekel (*Institute of Public Health (LÖGD), Germany*), Kirsi Nelimarkka, Kerttu Perttilä (*National Research and Development Centre for Welfare and Health (STAKES), Finland*), Nina Scagnetti (*Institute of Public Health of the Republic of Slovenia*), Martin Sprenger (*Medizinische Universität Graz, Austria*), Ingrid Stegeman (EuroHealthNet, Belgium), Marius Strička (*Kaunas University of Medicine*), Rudolf Welteke (*Institute of Public Health (LÖGD)*, Germany), Gareth Williams (*Cardiff University School of Social Sciences*) and Matthias Wismar (*European Observatory on Health Systems and Policies, Brussels*) (along with secondary contributors).

Contributors to individual country-specific case studies:

Case study 1: England
Katie Collins (*Opinion Leader Research*) and Lorraine Taylor (*National Institute for Health and Clinical Excellence*)

Case study 2: Italy
Roberta Siliquini (*Department of Public Health, University of Torino*), Nicola Nante (*Department of Public Health, University of Siena*) and Walter Ricciardi (*Institute of Hygiene, Catholic University of Sacred Heart*)

Case study 3: Lithuania
Marius Strička (*Kaunas University of Medicine*), Ingrida Zurlytė (*State Environmental Health Centre*) and Vilius Grabauskas (*Kaunas University of Medicine*)

Case study 4: The Netherlands
Janneke van Reeuwijk-Werkhorst and Loes van Herten
Netherlands Organisation for Applied Scientific Research (TNO)

Case study 5: Northern Ireland
Teresa Lavin and Owen Metcalfe
Institute of Public Health in Ireland

Case study 6: Slovenia
Mojca Gabrijelčič Blenkuš and Nina Scagnetti
Institute of Public Health of the Republic of Slovenia

Case study 7: Spain
Francisco Barroso (and Rosa Ferrera)
Técnicas de Salud, S.A.

Case study 8: Sweden
Ida Knutsson and Anita Linell
Swedish National Institute of Public Health

Case study 9: Wales
Eva Elliott, Alison Golby (*Cardiff Institute of Society, Health and Ethics, Cardiff University School of Social Sciences*) and Gareth Williams (*Cardiff University School of Social Sciences*)

Case study 10: Finland
Kirsi Nelimarkka, Tapani Kauppinen and Kerttu Perttilä
National Research and Development Centre for Welfare and Health (STAKES)

Case study 11: Germany
Rudolf Welteke, Thomas Classen, Odile Mekel, Rainer Fehr
Institute of Public Health (LÖGD)

Case study 12: Poland
Anicenta Bubak (*National Reference Centre on Environmental Health Impact Assessment, Institute for Ecology of Industrial Areas Katowice*) and Ewa Nowak (*Institute of Public Health Medical College, Jagiellonian University*)

Case study 13: Transport-related health effects in 6 countries (Austria, France, Malta, the Netherlands, Sweden, Switzerland)
Martin Sprenger and Ursula Püringer
Medizinische Universität Graz, Austria

Case study 14: Denmark
Gabriel Gulis
University of Southern Denmark, Unit of health promotion research

Case study 15: Hungary
Edit Eke
Semmelweis University Health Services Management Training Centre

Case study 16: Ireland
Teresa Lavin and Owen Metcalfe
Institute of Public Health in Ireland

Case study 17: Switzerland
Konrade von Bremen
Institute of Health Economics and Management (IEMS), University of Lausanne

Why research HIA? An introduction to the volume

Matthias Wismar, European Observatory on Health Systems and Policies

HIA as a decision-support tool

If it was a societal and political aim to avoid or minimize negative impacts on health, it would be necessary to feed information on the health impacts of a proposal and its alternatives into the decision-making process. One method would be the use of a decision-support tool such as HIA. There are many definitions of HIA – and the Gothenburg consensus is probably the best known among them (European Centre for Health Policy, 1999 (cit. Diwan et al., 2001)) – but as John Kemm argues in Chapter 1, most researchers would agree that HIA has two essential features (Kemm & Parry, 2004).

1. It is intended to support decision-making in choosing between options.

2. It does this by predicting the future consequences of implementing the different options.

HIA is seen as a universal decision-support tool, applicable at all political administrative levels. This is explored in detail in this volume. The case study of the assessment of a City Council's air quality action plan in Northern Ireland (Case study 5) shows its use on a local level. Use of HIA at regional level is demonstrated by the case study which utilizes the elements of HIA to determine the effects of air pollution in Ticino, Switzerland (Case study 17). A national-level HIA is demonstrated by the case study on the food production and nutrition impacts of Slovenia adopting the European Union's Common Agricultural Policy (Case study 6). Elements of HIA are being implemented at the supranational level as part of the European Commission's (EC) impact assessment; and on a much smaller level in an individual company's internal decision-making processes in Spain (Case study 7).

HIA is also seen as a universally applicable decision-support tool for the sectors concerned. This book explores sectoral case studies concerning agriculture, environment, land use, telecommunication, transport, urban planning and the workplace. Literature searches have identified HIAs on tax policies (Roscam Abbing, van Zoest & Varela Put, 2001), employment strategies (Haigh & Mekel, 2004), leisure and sport facilities (Thomson, Kearns & Petticrew, 2003) and foreign policy (Lee et al., 2007). HIA has also been seen as a decision-support tool sensitive to the determinants of health inequities (Barnes & Scott-Samuel, 2002; Fosse, 2006; Taylor et al., 2003; Simpson et al., 2005). Most HIAs have an explicit aim to profile the population affected by a proposal, for example, to identify vulnerable groups.

The assumed universal applicability and sensitivity towards inequities have attracted much attention within the research community. This can be seen by HIA's progress as a discipline (Kemm, 2005). The international literature on HIA is growing rapidly: theoretical, methodological and conceptual progress has been accompanied by fully fledged HIA reports and case studies. These include published country reports from Germany (Fehr, Mekel & Welteke, 2004), the Netherlands (Roscam Abbing, 2004; Varela Put et al., 2001) and the United Kingdom including Scotland (Douglas & Muirie, 2004) and Wales (Breeze, 2004). Many countries and subnational entities have developed HIA resources such as databases and websites, while others have embarked on capacity building. These initiatives have devised guidelines, tools and instruments; developed additional websites containing HIA databases, and made documents and tools available online. Some countries have developed successful HIA training courses and dedicated HIA units affiliated to, or integrated with, academic departments.

Various European governments have endorsed HIA; some have made explicit commitments by putting it on the political agenda. Some countries have included HIA in official policy papers and funded pilot projects. HIA has received support at supranational level too. The EC included aspects of human health in its directive on environmental impact assessment and health is an element of its internal impact assessment (Hübel & Hedin, 2003). The use of HIA was proposed in the EC's draft health strategy and endorsed by Member States and stakeholders. The World Health Organization (WHO) has supported HIA in the European Region, including it in the HEALTH 21 policy (WHO Regional Office for Europe, 1999). Additionally, various programmes and centres work to support the development. The 2005 update of WHO's Health for All lists HIA as a tool for implementing ethical governance (WHO Regional Office for Europe, 2005).

This introduction starts by explaining briefly the relevance of HIA with regard to health determinants, population health and health inequities. This is followed by a discussion of the social and economic health determinants and the role and potential of HIA as a decision-support tool. The motivation of the research is discussed by addressing some uncertainties about the usefulness of HIA in practice; the research objectives are derived from this. Finally, the book's structure is presented.

The link between health determinants, population health and health inequities

Health impact assessment is so important for addressing population health and health inequities because it tackles health determinants. It has become a common belief in Europe that health is determined largely by factors outside the health-care sector. A widely published model (Dahlgren & Whitehead, 1991; Dahlgren & Whitehead, 2006) describes five determinants of health:

1. biological factors such as age, sex and hereditary factors;

2. individual lifestyle factors such as eating and drinking habits, physical activity, smoking and alcohol consumption;

3. social and community networks;

4. living and working conditions such as agriculture and food production, education, work environment, unemployment, water and sanitation, health-care services and housing;

5. general socioeconomic, cultural and environmental conditions.

As health determinants often are interrelated and can build complex causal pathways when impacting on health (Kemm, 2006), they should not be viewed in isolation. For example, a lifestyle-related habit such as binge drinking may have been influenced, or even caused by, other determinants, the lack of a supportive social network, for example. Its lack may have been caused by poor living conditions (such as unemployment or residing in a deprived area) which, in turn, may have been influenced by general economic factors.

This lifestyle example also refers to the determinants of inequities in health (Dahlgren & Whitehead, 2006; Mackenbach, 2005; Mackenbach et al., 2004). There are a number of determinants of inequity in health. Social position in society (defined by education, occupation or economic resources) exerts a powerful influence on the type, magnitude and distribution of health risks experienced within different socioeconomic groups. In itself it is an important determinant of social inequities in health. Different levels of exposure contribute to the determinants of inequity in health too. Examples include exposure to chemical agents at the workplace, or housing close to busy roads, railway tracks or airports (Dahlgren & Whitehead, 2006).

Social and economic health determinants and decision-making

Those determinants more likely to be amenable to change from political decisions are known as the social and economic determinants of health. These contrast with biological determinants which are not altered so easily. Changes to social and economic determinants may be the result of decisions introducing, modifying or revoking policies, programmes or projects. Consequently, changes induced by political decision-making can result in changes to overall population health.

A decision's potential impact on the health of a population is a pressing problem for policy-makers, the affected population, developers and other stakeholders. Examples from this book may illustrate this. What will be the health impacts of the planned Berlin Brandenburg International airport (Case study 11); the proposed ecosystem revitalization to create a new damp zone in a rural area in Italy (Case study 2); or the erection of a mobile phone antenna on a school roof in Poland (Case study 12)? These projects are expected to affect social and economic determinants such as living, working or general environmental conditions. The expected increases in noise and pollution emissions, risk of infection for animals and humans, mosquito infestation and exposure to electromagnetic fields may impact on the health of the affected population. Even if not all of these impacts take place, the proposals cause concern and anxiety among the affected populations.

The same proposals may also have positive effects on working, living and general economic conditions, even producing positive health effects. The Berlin airport is likely to create new job opportunities in an area stricken with high unemployment rates; the damp zone is expected to develop into a recreational area for locals and might bring business opportunities for the local economy by attracting tourists; and the mobile phone antenna is expected to improve communication structures.

Decision-makers will face the situation that these impacts on health are distributed unevenly over different population groups. This introduces the determinants of health inequities. Winners and losers from changes in social and economic determinants may belong to different population groups. Those with new jobs at the airport are not necessarily those exposed to its nocturnal noise emissions. Those who enjoy the damp zone's wildlife are not necessarily those living in the immediate neighbourhood plagued by mosquitoes and noxious odours in summer. And those business people who benefit from the improved communication infrastructure will not necessarily work in offices located under the mobile phone antenna.

How useful is HIA in practice?

Some individual case studies and anecdotal evidence seem to suggest that HIA effectively supports the decision-making process. But it is difficult, if not impossible, to make comparisons as there are only a few case studies and various conceptual frameworks are used to analyse effectiveness. Often, an HIA's capacity to support the decision-making process is not analysed; in many cases it is arguable whether the impact assessment has been completely detached from the decision-making process. Recently, a more thorough and systematic approach was implemented by conducting a cost–benefit analysis of 15 HIAs. This study found that the benefits derived from the sample HIAs outweigh the cost of undertaking them, suggesting that HIA is cost-effective (O'Reilly et al., 2006). It has strengthened the argument that HIA is effective. However, issues of the universal applicability of HIA are not fully addressed, since all the HIAs in the sample came from England and 7 out of 15 cases focused on health care and health promotion.

From a more theoretical point of view it could be argued that the effectiveness of HIA must be limited. In the terminology of system theory, HIA could be seen as an attempt to impose its own system objectives on others. Why should education, transport and environment sectors be concerned with health? In certain win–win situations health and other sectors interact well, but there are conflicting system objectives too, for example, the liberties of a market economy in tobacco or alcohol industries (Sihto, Ollia & Koivusalo, 2006). The recent experiences of the Nordic countries gradually loosening their grip on alcohol-control policies have demonstrated that the free movement of goods, an economic objective, can conflict with health (Tigerstedt et al., 2006). Apart from the abstract language of system theory, those within a government's economic affairs department may be irritated by the health department's (perceived) intrusion into their remit. In fact, intersectoral collaboration has shown that health ministries usually act very cautiously or wait for good opportunities when trying to establish these links.

European countries share many common values, principles and ambitions. However, diversity is the key characteristic as implementation is highly context-dependent. This raises questions about HIA. Is it conceivable that one tool fits all countries? Conversely, given the institutional, political and economic differences across Europe, can all countries fit HIA? These doubts are reinforced by an apparently sluggish uptake of HIA in some parts of Europe. Apart from England, Wales and some of the Nordic countries, little activity has been reported in the international literature. The Netherlands, which institutionalized HIA on the national level, has gradually retrenched its activities so that HIA is confined to subnational level (Varela Put et al., 2001).

Research objectives and research strategy

This book is the outcome of a research project funded under the European Union Public Health Work Programme. The project's overall aim was to map the use of HIA, evaluate its effectiveness and identify factors for successful implementation. Within the context of the project, effectiveness refers to the capacity to support the decision-making process; decision-makers have taken adequate account of the results of the assessment.

The research strategy included mapping the use of HIA in Europe and an effectiveness analysis based on case studies. The research strategy was implemented by 21 teams from 19 countries.

In order to understand the analytical approach of this volume, it is essential to discuss briefly the conceptual framework of the effectiveness analysis detailed in Chapter 3, "The use of HIA across Europe". This distinguishes four types of effectiveness.

1. Direct effectiveness occurs if a decision is dropped or modified as a result of the HIA.

2. General effectiveness occurs if the assessment has been considered adequately by the decision-makers but does not result in modifications to the proposed decision.

3. Opportunistic effectiveness occurs if the HIA is conducted because it is assumed that it will support the proposed decision.

4. Ineffectiveness occurs when decision-makers do not take account of the assessment.

The effectiveness analysis is embedded in a second conceptual framework designed to identify factors that contribute to, or hinder, the effectiveness of HIA.

Structure of the book

The book is structured in five parts. Part I covers the essentials of the volume by presenting key issues, research and results. Chapter 1 addresses the question: what is HIA and why might it be useful? It introduces the key concepts of HIA and provides an overview on the key issues and the current debate. Chapter 2 introduces the conceptual frameworks and methodologies employed for the mapping of HIA across Europe and the effectiveness analysis. The chapter also provides a synthesis of the results of the mapping exercise and the effectiveness analysis, following the conceptual framework and the model presented earlier in the chapter. Building on this synthesis, the chapter then draws some conclusions on how to strengthen health in decision-making.

Part II of the book presents the European map of HIA. Chapter 3 provides an overview on the use of HIA across Europe. It addresses, for example, the frequency of HIA, the sectors concerned, the issues tackled and the political administrative levels. Chapter 4 addresses the role of governance, financing, resource generation and delivery in the implementation and institutionalization of HIA.

Part III presents a series of case studies on the effectiveness of HIA: from Italy, the Netherlands, Lithuania, Slovenia, Spain, Sweden and the United Kingdom (England, Wales and Northern Ireland). These cover a broad range of different sectors such as urban development (Case study 1; Case study 4), land use (Case study 2; Case study 9), transport (Case study 3), environment (Case study 5), agricultural policy (Case study 6) and the workplace (Case study 7).

HIA is not the only assessment that takes account of the health impact of decisions. There is discussion about whether health can be addressed more effectively by stand-alone HIAs or by integration within another, preferably obligatory, assessment. Part IV contributes to this debate by presenting three case studies in which health is integrated within other assessments in Finland, Germany and Poland. These cover the environmental and social impact assessment of land use (Case study 10), transport (Case study 11) and telecommunications (Case study 12).

The remaining case studies, in Part V, focus on using elements of HIA. These do not comply fully with the two key features of HIA described earlier but elements were employed either to test the feasibility of HIA or to develop an HIA implementation agenda. These case studies also show some effectiveness despite being largely detached from the immediate decision-making processes.

REFERENCES

European Centre for Health Policy (1999). Health impact assessment: main concepts and suggested approach. Gothenburg consensus paper, December 1999. In: Diwan V, et al., eds. *Health impact assessment: from theory to practice.* Gothenburg, Nordic School of Public Health, 2001:89–103.

Barnes R, Scott-Samuel A (2002). Health impact assessment and inequalities. *Revista Panamericana de Salud Pública [Pan American Journal of Public Health]*, 11(5/6):449–453.

Breeze C (2004). The experience of Wales. In: Kemm J, Parry J, Palmer S, eds. *Health impact assessment.* Oxford, Oxford University Press, 201–212.

Dahlgren G, Whitehead M (1991). *Policies and strategies to promote social equity in health.* Stockholm, Institute for Future Studies.

Dahlgren G, Whitehead M (2006). *Levelling up (part 2): a discussion paper on European strategies for tackling social inequities in health.* Copenhagen, WHO Regional Office for Europe.

Douglas M , Muirie J (2004). HIA in Scotland. In: Kemm J, Parry J, Palmer S, eds. *Health impact assessment.* Oxford, Oxford University Press, 191–200.

Fehr R, Mekel O, Welteke R (2004). HIA: the German perspective. In: Kemm J, Parry J, Palmer S, eds. *Health impact assessment.* Oxford, Oxford University Press, 253–264.

Fosse E (2006). *Social inequality in health impact assessment.* Oslo, Directorate for Health and Social Affairs.

Haigh F, Mekel O (2004). *Policy Health Impact Assessment for the European Union: Pilot Health Impact Assessment of the European Employment Strategy in Germany.* Brussels, European Commission.

Hübel M, Hedin A (2003). Developing health impact assessment in the European Union. *Bulletin of the World Health Organization,* 81(6):463–464.

Kemm J (2005). HIA – growth and prospects. *Environmental Impact Assessment Review,* 25(7–8):691–692.

Kemm J (2006). Health impact assessment and health in all policies. In: Ståhl T, et al., eds. *Health in all policies: prospects and potentials.* Helsinki, Ministry of Social Affairs and Health, 189–207.

Kemm J, Parry J (2004). What is HIA? Introduction and overview. In: Kemm J, Parry J, Palmer S, eds. *Health impact assessment.* Oxford, Oxford University Press, 1–13.

Lee K, Ingram A, Lock K, McInnes C (2007). Bridging health and foreign policy: the role of health impact assessments. *Bulletin of the World Health Organization,* 85(3):207–211.

Mackenbach JP (2005). *Health inequalities: Europe in profile.* London, Central Office of Information.

Mackenbach JP, et al. (2004). Health inequalities and HIA. In: Kemm J, Parry J, Palmer S, eds. *Health impact assessment.* Oxford, Oxford University Press, 25–37.

O'Reilly J, et al. (2006). *Cost–benefit analysis of health impact assessment.* London, Department of Health.

Roscam Abbing EW (2004). HIA and national policy in the Netherlands. In: Kemm J, Parry J, Palmer S, eds. *Health impact assessment.* Oxford, Oxford University Press, 177–189.

Roscam Abbing EW, van Zoest FF, Varela Put G (2001). Health impact assessment and intersectoral policy at national level in the Netherlands. In: Diwan V, et al., eds *Health impact assessment: from theory to practice.* Gothenburg, Nordic School of Public Health.

Sihto M, Ollia E, Koivusalo M (2006). Principles and challenges of health in all policies. In: Ståhl T, et al., eds. *Health in all policies: prospects and potentials.* Helsinki, Ministry of Social Affairs and Health, 3–20.

Simpson S, et al. (2005). Equity-focused health impact assessment: a tool to assist policy makers in addressing health inequalities. *Environmental Impact Assessment Review*, 25(7–8):772–782.

Taylor L, Gowman N, Quigley R. (2003) *Learning from practice bulletin: addressing inequalitiesthrough health impact assessment.* London, Health Development Agency (http://iaia. org/non_members/pubs_ref_material/Addressing%20Inequalities%20HIA%20pdf.pdf, accessed 14 August 2007).

Thomson S, Kearns A, Petticrew M (2003). Asssessing the health impact of local amenities: a qualitative study of contrasting experiences of local swimming pool and leisure provision in two areas of Glasgow. *Journal of Epidemiology and Community Health*, 57:663–667.

Tigerstedt C, et al. (2006). Health in alcohol policies: the European Union and its Nordic Member States. In: Kemm J, Parry J, Palmer S, eds. *Health impact assessment.* Oxford, Oxford University Press, 111–128.

Varela Put G, et al. (2001). *Experience with HIA at national policy level in the Netherlands. A case study.* Brussels, WHO Regional Office for Europe.

WHO Regional Office for Europe (1999). *Health 21: the Health for All policy framework for the WHO European Region.* Copenhagen, WHO Regional Office for Europe.

WHO Regional Office for Europe (2005). *The health for all policy framework for the WHO European Region: 2005 update.* Copenhagen, WHO Regional Office for Europe. Fifty-fifth session (http://www. euro.who.int/Document/RC55/edoc08.pdf, accessed 22 August 2007).

Part I
Health Impact Assessment: Key Issues, Research and Results

Chapter 1

What is HIA and why might it be useful?

John Kemm, West Midlands Public Health Observatory, Birmingham, United Kingdom

What is health impact assessment (HIA)?

The most widely quoted definition of HIA was produced at a meeting in Gothenburg organized by the World Health Organization (European Centre for Health Policy, 1999). It is "a combination of procedures, methods and tools by which a policy, programme or project may be judged as to its potential effects on the health of a population, and the distribution of those effects within the population."

More concisely, HIA has two essential features (Kemm & Parry, 2004).

1. It is intended to support decision-making in choosing between options.

2. It does this by predicting the future consequences of implementing the different options.

Some would add a third essential feature of HIA: stakeholder participation, involving the people affected by, or who have an interest in, a decision. This will be discussed later in the chapter.

Several reviews have discussed the purpose and methods of HIA, together with its strengths and weaknesses (Parry & Stevens, 2001; Morrison, Petticrew & Thomson, 2001; Mindell, Ison & Joffe, 2003; Joffe & Mindell, 2005; Kemm, 2006).

Related activities

Many other public-health activities share features with HIA but should be distinguished from it. The following definitions use intervention to cover any intended action including regulatory changes, provision of service, educational activity, construction of infrastructure and provision of welfare benefits.

Health needs assessment: systematic analysis of the health problems of a community with a view to determining the services or interventions required to remedy or prevent them.

Evaluation: systematic study of the effect of an intervention (or unplanned event such as a pollution incident). Evaluation usually involves observation and comparison of groups who experienced the intervention or event with groups who did not.

Monitoring and surveillance: systematic collection of information on aspects of a community's health in order to identify emerging health problems (or benefits). Monitoring may be part of evaluation.

Community development (with a health focus): process involving work with a community to increase their understanding of how local factors influence their health, and their ability and power to alter those factors to the benefit of the community. Frequently, community development leads to community action.

At times, all these activities have been described as HIA but none satisfies the definition of being linked to a specific decision and involving prediction. Early literature on HIA talked of prospective, concurrent and retrospective HIA. If prediction is an essential feature of HIA then it is tautological to call it prospective. Retrospective HIA (observing the effect of decisions already implemented) is no more than evaluation; concurrent HIA no more than monitoring. Therefore the terms prospective, concurrent and retrospective should no longer be used to qualify HIA (Morgan, 2003).

The purpose of HIA

From the definition of HIA it follows that it is intended to inform decision-makers by predicting the consequences of implementing different options, thereby enabling them to choose the option most beneficial for health and health equity. If there is participation then the HIA has a further purpose: to involve stakeholders in the decision and make the process more open.

HIA brings other benefits. It is extremely effective in encouraging cooperation between different agencies (for example health and local authorities). It increases awareness of health in the community and among decision-makers.

Application of HIA

Experience of HIA has been gathered in many European countries (Blau et al., 2006) as well as in Australia, New Zealand, Canada, south-east Asia and, recently, the United States of America. However, it is obligatory only in some countries which demand consideration of health impacts as a component of environmental impact assessment (EIA). To date it has been undertaken haphazardly, dependent on individual authorities' willingness to consider health, and the availability of HIA enthusiasts able to undertake assessments. Equally, there has been no consistent method or content. In some countries HIAs have focused on environmentally (noise and pollution) mediated health impacts; others have focused on participatory approaches and a broad view of health. However, the number of completed HIAs has risen steadily and many reports have been published.

While HIA is claimed to be applicable to projects, programmes and policies, it has been mostly applied to projects and city or regional policies rather than national-level policy (Lee et al., 2007). A unit to promote HIA policy was established in the Netherlands, another (now disbanded) was established in British Columbia in Canada. In England, policy preparation must include consideration of health but it is unclear whether this is carried out reliably.

How to perform an HIA

There are many different ways to carry out an HIA. One end of the spectrum is a brief, desk-based consideration involving three or four people for a few hours. The other is a prolonged consideration involving extensive literature searches; reanalysis of existing data; (possibly) collection of new primary data; and extensive consultation with stakeholders. This takes many months and involves many people.

There is no single correct method of HIA as it is applied to an enormous range of decisions, varying from international policy to very local projects, and an equally wide range of topics. The appropriate method varies according to the particular question under consideration. Generally, it is considered to have five stages: screening; scoping; assessment of impacts; reporting to decision-makers; and monitoring the consequences of implementation.

Screening indicates whether a decision is likely to have health consequences and whether an HIA is required. Scoping is used to plan the HIA by identifying the ways in which a decision could affect health; those who might be affected; how the impacts should be assessed; types of evidence; and resources to be used. Assessment of impacts is the main stage which clarifies the nature and size of the various impacts likely to arise under the different options. During recommendations and reporting, assessors seek to identify and report to decision-makers on recommendations to prevent or reduce negative impacts and enhance positive impacts for each option. Finally, the situation is monitored when an option (which could be "do nothing") is implemented.

Prediction

The claim that HIA is useful rests on its ability to predict the consequences of different options. It is therefore reasonable to ask HIA practitioners if their predictions are more reliable than those of crystal-ball gazing or any other method.

Logic paths are key to HIA prediction. These set out what will be changed by the implementation of possible decisions and how these changes will impact on health (Joffe & Mindell, 2006). A decision may be expected to change various intermediate factors (such as employment, social capital, air quality, built and natural environment) which, in turn, produce changes in specified health outcomes.

A preliminary logic diagram should be part of the scoping stage, serving to clarify assumptions, highlight important causal mechanisms and reveal knowledge gaps. The first step in the logic path nearly always requires knowledge other than public health. For example, traffic engineers to predict changes in traffic flows; economists to predict employment and income changes; or chemical engineers to predict flue emissions and plume distributions. Public health expertise assesses how these predicted changes will impact on health. The logic diagram is also very helpful at the recommendation stage as it demonstrates the paths to positive or negative impacts.

An HIA based on epidemiological/toxicological reasoning would go on to estimate the levels of different hazards which people will experience (exposure) and their effects (dose response curve) in order to assess the likely impacts on health. However, often the necessary exposure and dose response information is unobtainable or the causal mechanisms are understood insufficiently to make this method possible.

An HIA based on sociological reasoning draws prediction information from what those affected think is likely to happen. This takes account of their fears, perceptions and experience of living in a community which is likely to be affected (Elliott & Williams, 2004).

Participation

The place of participation is hotly debated within HIA. Many regard it as an essential feature and would not accept any process that does not include it. Others regard participation as one of many tools available, extremely helpful in some contexts but not in others (Parry & Wright, 2003).

The case for participation rests on five main purposes. Firstly, residents understand better than anyone what it is like to live in their environment and therefore are essential sources of information on how it might be changed. Secondly, it can be argued that people have a right to see how decisions that affect them are being made. Thirdly, it can be argued that people have a right to take part in decisions that affect them. Fourthly, where a decision is under dispute, conflict resolution may be helped by involvement in a process which examines systematically the case for and against. Lastly, participation in an HIA will increase a community's knowledge and ability to control things that influence their health.

While these are powerful arguments for participation, closer scrutiny is needed before requiring it to be a part of every HIA. For example, an expert is likely to provide a more accurate answer to a question about how many micrograms of dioxin per year a process will emit. However, the acceptability of this technical answer involves a value judgement which puts a much stronger case for participative methods. Also, if participation is appropriate for local projects, how can it be applied to decisions affecting thousands or tens of thousands in projects involving whole cities or regions? All those affected cannot participate directly so involvement must be through representation. Participation in HIA of national-level policy is even more problematic. Can national policy be developed without secrecy in the early stages and can direct participation add anything to representative democracy?

Participation may be attempted by asking people to sit on the HIA steering group, conducting interviews or surveys, or by holding focus groups or public meetings. Yet each of these raises theoretical as well as logistical problems. Who decides who will participate? Often, HIA assessors argue that they are listening to the voice of the weak and voiceless. This is laudable but what is their mandate to decide who will represent the various interest groups in the community? Why are some groups represented and others not? Professionals who work in the community (such as community nurses or social workers) may argue that they represent these communities, but is that acceptable? Is anyone consulted on who will represent them? All too often practices which claim to be participative appear very paternalistic.

HIA and decision-making

There is increasing consideration of how HIA can be most useful to decision-makers and of the barriers to its use (Lock & McKee, 2005; Davenport, Mathers & Parry, 2006). Early diagrams of HIA showed assessment and decision-making as part of a single process, with those who undertook the HIA also making the decision. This happens sometimes but generally is not true. Following the model of policy appraisal or EIA, those carrying out an appraisal or assessment are asked to advise the decision-makers, not make a decision on their behalf. HIA is a decision-support rather than a decision-making tool. It could be argued that the health impact assessor should be an impartial adviser rather than an advocate.

This point is contested strongly. Some consider that the assessor should be a forceful advocate for public health, strongly favouring those options that they believe will increase health, sustainability and equity (Scott-Samuel & O'Keefe, 2007). This changes their role from assessor to would-be decision-maker. Frequently, impartial assessment demonstrates that the health impacts of one option are much more favourable than any other. In such a case it is probably more effective to let the assessment speak for itself. If different options show very similar health impacts, it is necessary to question why any one of them is preferred. Little is gained by attempting to be both advocate and assessor; rather, it raises questions about impartiality.

Evaluation

HIA evaluation seeks to determine whether an HIA has led to a better decision. This differs from evaluation of the decision that it was meant to inform, which seeks to determine whether the implemented decision affected health outcomes. It is hard to find evidence that an HIA has had a beneficial effect on a decision. An exploration of decision-makers' perceptions probably is the best that can be achieved. Do they feel that the HIA was useful? How did it influence their decision-making? And how would their decision have differed without an HIA?

Process evaluation is also useful to show that an HIA's timing and content were appropriate and likely to have influenced the final decision. Time may reveal the accuracy of the predictions for chosen and implemented options, but not for those which were not implemented (the counterfactuals). Once again, process evaluation can show whether the methods used were thorough and likely to have produced an accurate prediction. The extent to which those in the affected community felt involved in the decision process can be determined through interviews and surveys; examination of the process will reveal the thoroughness of the attempt to achieve participation (Parry & Kemm, 2005).

Most evidence that HIA is effective comes from anecdote and case history. While this is far from a rigorous evaluation, there is a general impression that decision-makers have found HIAs helpful in many cases.

Health in other assessments

Advocates consider that a large and increasing number of decisions would benefit from HIA. However, decision-makers may be reluctant to engage, as this is only one of several assessments that they may be urged to undertake: EIA; sustainability assessment (SA); and checking their decisions against a wide range of cross-cutting issues such as the implications for gender, ethnic minorities, law and order, rural communities and so on. It is little wonder that suggestions for further impact assessment are unwelcome. The solution is to seek ways of reducing the burden on decision-makers rather than argue that health issues are more deserving of attention.

Many of the questions explored in HIA are common to other assessments. Health impacts are nearly always mediated through other impacts, for example, health can be considered as part of an EIA. This has not been covered well to date but if decision-makers reject EIA reports which lack information on health the practice will improve. Strategic environmental assessment (SEA), introduced under European law, requires that population and health should be assessed alongside other environmental aspects (Williams & Fisher, 2007).

Some organizations are experimenting with integrated impact assessment, which attempts to combine all aspects of impact assessments within a single process. By definition, integrated impact assessments cover more topics but in less detail than a single impact assessment. However, a limited assessment is better than none. The goal of all activities should be always to consider health in public decision-making. It is immaterial whether this is achieved by a process called HIA or by some other name.

What skills are required for HIA?

Numerous skills are required to undertake an HIA. Project management skills identify the various elements in the process; to decide the order and time scale in which they must be undertaken; and to ensure timely completion to the quality required. Negotiating skills ensure that the assessment fits the agendas of both the decision-makers and the assessment team. Team-working skills draw together the contributions of experts in different disciplines with stakeholders. Community skills engage with those affected by a proposal and facilitate participation, as does an ability to listen actively, draw out and see the meaning in lay knowledge. Research skills assist the collection and understanding of data on the current health state of the relevant population, and literature searches for information on links between intermediate variables and health. Advice and help from experts in other disciplines may be required to analyse how the options will affect intermediate variables such as income, employment, exposure to pollutants and so on.

This list makes clear that HIA is neither difficult nor overly scientific. The key requirements are robust common sense, an ability to pull together disparate elements to form a big picture and a capacity to persuade different people to work in cooperation. These skills are not peculiar to public health specialists; until recently most were carried out by people who claimed no special HIA expertise. It is not correct to assert that HIA requires rare skills and a new profession of health impact assessors. We should be persuading many people that they are capable of performing HIA, promoting confidence by helping them to acquire extra skills and encouraging new projects.

It has been argued that HIA has a special value set. The Gothenburg consensus (European Centre for Health Policy, 1999) lists key values: openness, equity, sustainability and ethical use of evidence. Others have urged that HIA practitioners should be passionate campaigners for justice. However, the simple values required are honesty combined with rigorous analysis.

Capacity building

How is it possible to meet the requirement for HIA, or at least many more systematic considerations of health consequences? Only a few people are currently undertaking HIA, mostly as a minor part of their work. It is unlikely to be possible to produce a workforce of specialized health impact assessors large enough to undertake all the work required. Also, as discussed above, a specialized workforce would be wasteful and unnecessary.

Capacity can be increased by encouraging many more people in managerial and policy posts to undertake their own HIAs. Health impact assessors will have been truly successful when many of those outside the community feel able to carry out these assessments. At government level, HIA should be part of the routine policy-making procedure undertaken by all ministries rather than the special responsibility of the health ministry. The practice of HIA is discouraged by the misconception that it is a very time-consuming activity that requires arcane knowledge and by uncertainty over how to set about it. These barriers could be reduced by establishing HIA support centres at national or regional level to provide advice and guidance.

There is a strong case for requiring consideration of health in all public decisions although, as argued before, this could be part of an integrated assessment rather than a separate HIA. Equally, consideration of health should be an obligatory element in the development of all new legislation. Such a requirement would necessitate measures to increase HIA capacity as numbers would increase.

Resourcing HIA

Discussion of HIA capacity inevitably leads to questions about resources. These have not been addressed properly in most HIAs performed to date: resources, professional time and incidental expenses have been found within the assessing organizations. In some cases, the decision-makers have contributed towards costs but, generally, these have fallen far short of full business costing.

If HIA becomes part of the routine decision-making process there will be no need to identify separate budget lines. However, the resource implications (chiefly additional time) will have to be factored into every department's work plan. HIA support centres would require separate funding, most logically from central departments of health or public-health funds. The cost of HIA has not been researched properly but preliminary enquiries suggest that the benefits far exceed the costs (Atkinson & Cooke, 2005; O'Reilly et al., 2006).

Where public permission for a proposal (for example, planning permission for building; industrial process operating licence application) requires an HIA, as for any other permission requirements, the proposer should pay. This is well established for EIA and could apply equally well to HIA. However, it is important that the assessor remains accountable to, and works for, the relevant regulatory authority.

HIA governance

If HIA is to be useful it must be performed honestly, impartially and competently. Yet procedures to ensure this are poorly developed. It has been suggested that health impact assessors should be accredited and, perhaps, required to attend prescribed courses. This raises three objections: (1) all too often, formal accreditation is no guarantee of competence; (2) the development of a profession excludes others from undertaking HIA; (3) most seriously, the attempt to define best practice risks preventing change in what should be a rapidly developing field.

Openness is the best protection against unsatisfactory practice so all HIA reports should be freely available to the public. Where HIA is part of a process regulated by law (for example planning permissions in the United Kingdom or strategic environmental assessment (SEA)), faulty HIAs will be subject to legal challenge. In other contexts, public scrutiny will identify a biased HIA that has based its conclusions on unsound reasoning or neglected important causal paths. Health ministries can usefully encourage good practice within all parts of government performing a developmental rather than a regulatory role. HIA governance should focus on the quality of the product rather than the qualifications of the assessors.

Equity and HIA

Equity – a fair distribution of benefits – is a policy goal in most countries. Most decisions have winners who benefit and losers who suffer harm or, at least, benefit less. For example, where there is an out-of-town shopping centre those with cars would benefit, those without would experience negative impacts. The construction of a waste incinerator has more negative impacts for those living nearby but positive impacts for those living further away or, perhaps, at alternative disposal sites.

HIA can contribute to health equity by identifying those likely to experience positive and negative impacts and what those impacts should be. It may be able to recommend modifications to a proposal in order to reduce negative impacts or achieve a more equitable distribution. However, the final judgement on the fairness of a particular distribution of impacts should rest with a democratically accountable decision-maker not a health impact assessor.

Conclusion

This short review presents a personal view. Many of those who practise HIA may disagree with some of the author's conclusions but it is hoped that they agree that these are the issues which need debate. HIA is a young and developing discipline that shows much promise for helping public decision-makers to make healthier choices.

REFERENCES

Atkinson P, Cooke A (2005). Developing a framework to assess costs and benefits of health impact assessment. *Environmental Impact Assessment Review*, 25:791–798.

Blau J, et al. (2006). The use of health impact assessment across Europe. In: Ståhl T, et al., eds. *Health in all policies: prospects and potentials.* Helsinki, Ministry of Social Affairs and Health, 209–230.

Davenport C, Mathers J, Parry J (2006). Use of health impact assessment in incorporating health considerations in decision-making. *Journal of Epidemiology and Community Health*, 60:196–201.

Elliot E, Williams G (2004). Developing a civic intelligence: local involvement in HIA. *Environmental Impact Assessment Review*, 24:231–244.

European Centre for Health Policy (1999). *Health impact assessment: main concepts and suggested approach. Gothenburg consensus paper.* Copenhagen, WHO Regional Office for Europe.

Joffe M, Mindell J (2005). Health impact assessment. *Occupational and Environmental Medicine*, 62:907–912.

Joffe M, Mindell J (2006). Complex causal process diagrams for analysing the health impacts of policy interventions. *American Journal of Public Health*, 96:473–479.

Kemm J (2006). Health impact assessment and health in all policies. In: Ståhl T, et al., eds. *Health in all policies: prospects and potentials.* Helsinki, Ministry of Social Affairs and Health, 189–207.

Kemm J, Parry J (2004). What is HIA? Introduction and overview. In: Kemm J, Parry J, Palmer S. eds. *Health impact assessment: concepts, theory, techniques and applications.* Oxford, Oxford University Press, 1–13.

Lee K, et al. (2007). Bridging health and foreign policy: the role of health impact assessment. *Bulletin of the World Health Organization*, 85:207–211.

Lock K, McKee M (2005). Health impact assessment: assessing opportunities and barriers to intersectoral health improvement in an expanded European Union. *Journal of Epidemiology and Community Health*, 59:356–360.

Mindell J, Ison E, Joffe M (2003). A glossary for health impact assessment. *Journal of Epidemiology and Community Health*, 57:647–651.

Morgan RK (2003). Health impact assessment: the wider context. *Bulletin of the World Health Organization*, 81:390.

Morrison DS, Petticrew M, Thomson H (2001). Health impact assessment and beyond. *Journal of Epidemiology and Community Health*, 55:219–220.

O'Reilly J, et al. (2006). *Cost–benefit analysis of health impact assessment.* York, York Health Economics Consortium (http://www.dh.gov.uk/en/Publicationsandstatistics/Publications/ PublicationsPolicyAndGuidance/DH_063021, accessed 22 August 2007).

Parry J, Kemm J (2005). Criteria for use in evaluation of health impact assessments. *Public Health*, 119:1122–1129.

Parry J, Stevens A (2001). Prospective health impact assessment: pitfalls, problems and possible ways forward. *BMJ*, 323:1177–1182.

Parry J, Wright J (2003). Community participation in health impact assessments: intuitively appealing but practically difficult. *Bulletin of the World Health Organization*, 81:388.

Scott-Samuel A, O'Keefe E (2007). Health impact assessment, human rights and global public policy: a critical appraisal. *Bulletin of the World Health Organization*, 85:212–217.

Williams C, Fisher P (2007). *Draft guidance on health in strategic environmental assessment* (consultation document). London, Department of Health.

Chapter 2
Is HIA effective? A synthesis of concepts, methodologies and results

Matthias Wismar, Julia Blau and Kelly Ernst
European Observatory on Health Systems and Policies

Introduction

The "Effectiveness of health impact assessment" project[1] was carried out by 21 research teams from 19 countries.[2] The project started in 2004 and was concluded in 2007. The overall aim of the project was to map the use of health impact assessment (HIA), evaluate its effectiveness and identify the determinants for its successful implementation. Effectiveness in the context of this project referred to the capacity to influence the decision-making process and to be taken into account adequately by the decision-makers. The project had four specific objectives:

---

[1] The project was conducted with the financial assistance of the European Community (EC) in the framework of the Public Health Work Programme (Grant Agreement 2003101). The views expressed herein are those of the authors and can therefore in no way be taken to reflect the official opinion of the EC.

[2] The project was led by the European Observatory on Health Systems and Policies, and included as partners and national coordinators EuroHealthNet; National Institute for Health and Clinical Excellence (NICE, formerly Health Development Agency (HDA)), United Kingdom; Institute of Hygiene, Catholic University of the Sacred Heart, Italy; Institute of Public Health, Ireland; Institut za varovanje zdravjaa Republike Slovenije, Slovenia; Jagiellonian University, Institute of Public Health, Poland; Landesinstitut für den Öffentlichen Gesundheitsdienst NRW, Germany; National Institute of Public Health, Sweden; Semmelweiss University Budapest Health Services Management Training Centre, Hungary; National Research and Development Centre for Welfare and Health (STAKES), Finland; Técnicas de Salud SA, Spain; TNO Prevention and Health, the Netherlands; University of Southern Denmark; Wales Centre for Health, United Kingdom; WHO Collaborating Centre on Health and Psychosocial and Psychobiological Factors; Trnava University, Faculty of Health Care and Social Work, Department of Hygiene and Epidemiology, Slovakia; Directorate-General of Health (National Coordinator), Portugal; Medical University of Graz (National Coordinator), Austria; Institute of Health Economics and Management (National Coordinator), Switzerland; Kaunas Medical University (National Coordinator), Lithuania; Ministry of Health (National Coordinator), Malta.

Table 2.1 *Comparison of task 1 and task 2 by selected features*

	Mapping exercise	*Effectiveness analysis*
Definition of HIA effectiveness	"Open"	"Three dimensions of effectiveness with specific characteristics"
Methodology employed	Literature review using a detailed template (aggregated or global data)	Interviews (single case)
Key concepts	• terminology and definitions • HIA systems • practices • other assessments	• effectiveness of HIA • factors that facilitate or hinder effectiveness
Style	Descriptive	Analytical (causalities)
Outcome	European map of HIA	Case studies and analytical chapters

1. to map the use of HIA in European Union (EU) Member States;
2. to map the use of other impact assessment methodologies that have included health;
3. to develop a set of indicators to measure the implementation of HIA;
4. to assess the factors that enable or hinder the implementation of HIA, including the institutional, organizational and cultural contexts as well as the decision-making process.

This chapter synthesizes the concepts, methodologies and research results from the project. It is based on a mapping exercise and an effectiveness analysis implemented through 17 case studies included in this volume. The mapping exercise and the effectiveness analysis complement each other, and an overview on the differences between them is provided in Table 2.1.

The mapping exercise looked into the use, implementation and institutionalization of HIA across Europe and captured HIAs at the national, regional and local levels using a questionnaire and individual HIA fact sheets. It also explored the role of health in other assessments, such as environmental impact assessment (EIA) and social impact assessment (SIA). In addition, especially for countries with little experience in HIA, trials and activities were included in the research that used elements of HIA.

The purpose of the effectiveness analysis was to explore the effectiveness of HIA and health in other assessments in terms of their capacity to influence or modify a pending decision. The case studies also explored factors that contribute to their effectiveness. Results were taken from 17 case studies from 16 countries which include 9 HIAs, 3 other assessments that include a health component (EIA, SIA) and 5 case studies that, although not dealing with HIA in the strict sense of the definition, do use elements of HIA. Table 2.2 gives an

Table 2.2 *Case studies by sector, country and topic*

Transport

Austria, France, Malta, Netherlands, Sweden, Switzerland	Transport-related health effects in a transnational project	Case study 13
Germany	Berlin Brandenburg International (BBI) Airport construction	Case study 11
Republic of Ireland	Testing HIA methodology in the transport sector	Case study 16
Sweden	Reconstruction of Route 73	Case study 8
Switzerland	Air pollution exposure across the Alps	Case study 17

Urban planning

England	King's Cross area renovation	Case study 1
Finland	Land-use planning for a proposed residential area	Case study 10
Hungary	Obstacle-free environment for the disabled	Case study 15
Lithuania	Impacts of the Klaipeda National Seaport	Case study 3
Netherlands	Restructuring an industrial area into a residential area	Case study 4

Agriculture

Italy	Wet zone creation	Case study 2
Slovenia	Common Agricultural Policy	Case study 6

Environment

Northern Ireland	City Council's Air Quality Action Plan	Case study 5
Wales	Remediation of a landfill refuse site	Case study 9

Industry

Spain	Workplace smoking restriction policy	Case study 7

Infrastructure

Poland	Erection of a mobile phone base station antenna	Case study 12

Nutrition

Denmark	6-per-day programme: diet and cancer	Case study 14

overview of the case studies included in this book, showing the range of sectors in which HIA is utilized; Box 2.1 shows the methods behind the research and analysis involved; and Box 2.2 explains how the use and implementation of HIA were researched.

Box 2.1 *How the effectiveness of HIA and health in other assessments was researched and analysed*

The key methodology was interviews conducted with 3–6 people involved in the chosen HIA, complemented by the available literature, including grey literature. The HIA was chosen on the grounds of three criteria: it had to be included in the mapping exercise; it needed to have some stakeholder or community involvement; and had to have been recently completed. The interviews were supported by a resource package containing a conceptual paper, a user guide, interview questions, a case study template and an informed consent form. The conceptual paper was written on the basis of a literature review. External advice was sought for specifying the interview methodologies. The resource package was peer reviewed, pre tested and modified accordingly. The interviewers were trained in the use of the resource package via telephone conferences with 3–5 participants each. Interviews with decision-makers, stakeholders and members of the community involved in the HIA were conducted between February and May 2006. Early drafts of the case studies were reviewed and discussed by the project's steering group and were peer reviewed by two external experts.

Box 2.2 *How the use and implementation of HIA were researched*

The mapping exercise was based on 19 domestic literature reviews conducted by national project coordinators. The literature reviews also included grey literature. In order to facilitate systematic comparison, a questionnaire was designed, peer reviewed, pre tested and employed to abstract the data gathered by the literature search and to bring them into a common format. Instructions were posted to specify the role of the literature review, the design of the questionnaire, the search strategy and the use of the questionnaire. The questionnaire was divided into four parts: (1) terminology and general issues; (2) HIA systems; (3) fact sheets of individual HIAs; (4) health in other assessments. The search covered a period of 15 years from 1 January 1990 to 31 December 2004. The national level was searched comprehensively and this was complemented by searching one reference region and one reference locality for each country.

This chapter goes on to provide a synopsis of the results, concepts and methodologies on which these insights are based. The chapter starts by giving the reader a synthesis of the effectiveness analysis, covering types, magnitude and dimensions of effectiveness, the universal applicability of HIA, limits to the effectiveness of HIA and factors contributing to the effectiveness of HIA. This is followed by an overview of the results of the mapping exercise.

Is HIA effective?

Types of effectiveness

HIA can be effective as demonstrated by the individual HIA case studies included in this volume. According to the effectiveness analysis, in almost all of the 17 case studies, HIA proved to be effective in some way. An example of a case study that shows HIA as not directly effective is the Hungarian case study on an obstacle-free environment. The deadline for creating obstacle-free environments in all public buildings was 1 January 2005. However, due to delays, the pilot HIA was completed one year after the law came into effect. Advanced drafts therefore had no influence on the current legislation.

This key result has to be understood in connection with the common conceptual framework of the effectiveness analysis which included the definition of four different types of effectiveness.

The first type, **direct effectiveness**, refers to cases in which the HIA has contributed to a modification in the pending decision. This volume has many examples. In England, the King's Cross HIA was most directly effective in terms of health (Case study 1). The decision not to allow 24-hour working at King's Cross Central and the ensuing health benefits to the community were attributed directly to the Primary Care Trust's evidence at the planning enquiry. In addition, the problems identified with emergency planning and the subsequent changes in the planning proposals were attributed directly to the HIA. In the Finnish case study, direct health effectiveness can be seen in that certain traffic-planning arrangements were changed due to noise and safety implications (Case study 10). These solutions aimed to diminish the weaknesses and adverse effects of the plan.

General effectiveness, the second type, comprises cases where the results of the HIA have been taken into account adequately by the decision-makers but did not result in modification of the pending decision. For example, in the case studies from England, the Netherlands and Northern Ireland (Case studies 1, 4 and 5), sources were quoted stating that the HIA had created stronger health consciousness of decision-makers. According to the interviewees, for those involved, it brought about greater understanding of the links between the wider determinants of health and particular measures, and the health of the population. It was also felt that there has been a lasting effect which will contribute to healthy decision-making in the future.

Opportunistic effectiveness, the third type, can be seen when the HIA "seems to have" an effect on the decision, but in fact, the HIA was only initialized because it was expected to support a preferred policy option. While the outcomes in terms of health gains may be positive, it remains arguable as to whether the HIA was exploited on the grounds that the results were predictably in line with the dominant political force. It was difficult to find an HIA among the case studies which matched this type of effectiveness. This does not mean that this type of effectiveness does not exist. As explained, the results of the HIAs detailed in these case studies should not be overgeneralized. In the remediation of a landfill refuse site in Wales (Case study 9), the participatory approach of the HIA in order to resolve a long-lasting conflict was much more important than the modification of the pending decision.

The fourth type, **no effectiveness**, comprises all cases which do not fit into any of the above categories.

These types were defined on the basis of a matrix (see Table 2.3).

The effectiveness of HIA against health outcomes has purposely not been measured. Dismissing health outcomes as an analytical yardstick for the effectiveness analysis was not just based on the methodological difficulties that such an analysis would face. The long latency of health effects, the changing composition of the affected population and the difficulties in controlling and adjusting for confounders would make an outcome-based effectiveness analysis very difficult, if not impossible (Kemm & Parry, 2004; Wismar, 2005). The choice to conceptualize HIA as a decision-support tool was based on the assumption that scientific evidence cannot substitute decisions made for political reasons. In addition, other sectors may have different objectives which cannot easily be traded off for health objectives. Decision-makers sometimes chose the unhealthy decision, even when they are fully informed of the health consequences, because they feel that other sectoral values are equally, if not more, important.

Although according to the case studies the effectiveness of HIA seems quite clear cut, it has to be interpreted with great care as the aim was to refute the (null) hypothesis that HIA was ineffective. Therefore, any generalization should be avoided. Indeed, the case studies build by no means a representative sample, as only 17 cases from 15 countries were analysed. Nothing can be said about the effectiveness of all the others in these countries. Moreover, the research teams were purposely asked to choose HIAs for analyses which were assumed to have some potential for effectiveness.

In addition to the case studies on HIA and health in other assessments, five cases studies were included in the volume employing elements of HIA, although they were not connected to a pending decision. The authors, however, demonstrated that they were effective in terms of changing the context, leading in some cases to political action, and paving the way for further HIA activity.

Table 2.3 *Four types of effectiveness*

		Modification of pending decisions according to health/equity/community aspects and inputs	
		Yes	No
Health/equity/ community adequately acknowledged	Yes	*Direct effectiveness* • HIA-related changes in the decision • due to the HIA the project was dropped • decision was postponed	*General effectiveness* • reasons provided for not following HIA recommendations • health consequences are negligible or positive • HIA has raised awareness among policy-makers
	No	*Opportunistic effectiveness* • the decision would have been made anyway	*No effectiveness* • the HIA was ignored • the HIA was dismissed

Magnitude of effectiveness

Another key result of the research is that the magnitude of the influence of HIA on the pending decision varies greatly. The EIA of the BBI Airport had massive impacts on the development of the airport. It imposed a night flight ban, which diminished the airport's chances to attract traffic from Frankfurt, Munich and Vienna acting either as a hub for a major airline or a connection to eastern Europe. Without the additional traffic, the proposed airport may turn out to be oversized. On the other hand, there are examples, such as the HIA case study on the National Seaport development in Lithuania, which suggest that the HIA had very little effect on the core of the proposed decision (Case study 3). Its effect was rather to introduce additional noise protection in order to avoid the worst health impacts on the local residents. In summary, all the HIAs analysed in the case studies modified certain aspects of the pending decision but not a single project or development was completely withdrawn because of the HIA.

A further key result, rather unexpectedly, shows that some projects are so complex that they entail a large number of discrete decisions. This implies that the assessment may have different types of effectiveness working in parallel. Most case studies have indicated both direct and general effectiveness. For example, as described in the Finnish case study (Case study 10), there is direct health effectiveness since some traffic planning arrangements were changed based on noise and safety implications. There is also general health effectiveness, since discussion about recreational areas and sports facilities was brought to the forefront during the SIA negotiations.

Dimensions of effectiveness

The literature review, on which the conceptual framework was based, showed that HIA can be effective in various ways. The project identified three major dimensions of effectiveness: health effectiveness, equity effectiveness and community effectiveness (see Figure 2.1).

A key dimension of most HIAs is to avoid negative and strengthen positive health effects, but also the distribution of the health impacts is a highly relevant dimension of HIA effectiveness (Mackenbach et al., 2004). Equity effectiveness played a role in some case studies, but equity was rarely a distinctive issue in the modification of the decision. In the Finnish SIA on the land-use planning for a proposed residential area, the children's interests were taken into account in the city planning. The school playgrounds were preserved, thus improving recreational possibilities in the Kortepohja area, even though it meant an increase in the planning costs. The decision not to allow 24-hour working, as a result of the English HIA on the King's Cross area renovation (Case study 1), was seen as being equity effective as it affected the most economically disadvantaged members of the local community who lived in an estate very close to the construction work. In addition, groups such as homeless people, drug users and sex workers were included on an equal footing with other community members, because no one could deny their right to good health. In the Spanish HIA on the smoking restriction in the workplace policy (Case study 7), the equity aspect of the policy was assured by the heterogeneity of stakeholders in the working group that defined the key elements of the policy; the possibility for policy-receivers to participate directly in the decision-making (by means of the survey); and the equitable distribution of restrictions and enforcement across all job categories.

In the debate on HIA, the role of the community is frequently discussed. This refers to participatory issues ranging from transparency of decision-making to empowerment (Elliott, Williams & Rolfe, 2004; Elliott & Williams, 2004; Wright, Parry & Mathers, 2005). Many examples can be drawn from the case studies contained in this volume. In England, the fact that the HIA was in some part prompted by the actions of community members points to direct community effectiveness. The HIA conducted in Northern Ireland on the City Council's Air Quality Action Plan (Case study 5) shows clear links between suggestions made at community workshops and actions outlined in the final Action Plan. The company-based HIA in Spain included a strong community element as well, as the community's interests were acknowledged adequately in the decision-making process. The pending decision was modified, or even defined, by taking account of the opinions, interest,

Figure 2.1 *Conceptual framework effectiveness analysis*

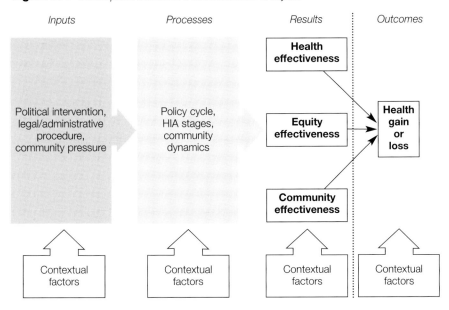

preferences or wishes of the employees. The company managers considered direct participation of the policy-receivers in the decision-making process to be a prerequisite for implementing the smoke-free policy (even granting them power to veto the initiative). In the HIA conducted in the Republic of Ireland (Case study 16), a strong community aspect was identified as well. The community was involved throughout the process, represented in the steering group and consulted through local groups. Community-based issues and decisions also featured strongly in the recommendations.

Some case studies have also reported positive effects on administration and policy-making. For example, the Slovenian HIA on the CAP (Lock et al., 2004) (Case study 6) was considered to be effective in the sense that it helped develop new communication links between the ministries responsible for food, nutrition and health issues. An important side-effect was the development of the ability to understand the positions and arguments of both sides, and identify common interests. Following discussions on the HIA, the health and agricultural sectors agreed on some common policy areas to support and implement in Slovenia after accession to the EU, such as the future interest in rural development policy.

In the Welsh case study (Case study 9), the HIA had an organizational impact by investing in staff skills which could be utilized in future assessments. The Finnish SIA activated cooperation and enhanced communication between various administrative areas, increasing the ability to take action and reach agreements, and made the actors commit to the planning process. In the Republic of Ireland, all respondents highlighted organizational effectiveness as a positive outcome of the HIA process. The council respondent emphasized the benefits of gaining insight into other organizations' work: "Working with other agencies and learning what others are doing was informative and effective. I became aware of what Health Promotion was doing in schools and we were doing similar work on road safety and walking or cycling to school. But if it was done together maybe we could have a more coordinated approach."

Universal applicability

Another key result of the effectiveness analysis is that HIA can be employed universally. The HIAs were effective across all countries. As Table 2.2 shows, the case studies covered a broad range of sectors and a considerably diverse range of issues.

The case studies also provided evidence that HIA can be effective on different levels, as seen in Table 2.4. However, this analysis also has to be interpreted with great care. Federalism, decentralization, deconcentration and devolution have brought about a large variety of institutional settings (Bankauskaite, Dubois & Saltman, 2007) which are not equivalent in international comparison. In some cases, joint decision-making is stretched over various levels, as in the German federal system, for example (Busse & Riesberg, 2004).

To make it even more complex, the match between the competent political administrative level and the level at which health impacts are expected may differ. In some cases, a national HIA is aiming at nationwide impacts, such as the Danish diet and cancer HIA (Case study 14) or the Slovenian HIA (Case study 6) on the Common Agricultural Policy (CAP). In other cases, a national assessment is looking at impacts at regional or local levels, such as the BBI Airport EIA (Case study 11) or the Swiss transport HIA (Case study 17).

The universal applicability of HIA, as demonstrated by the case studies, does not imply that context is not important. On the contrary, the case studies demonstrate that context is highly relevant when realizing the full potential of HIA.

Limits to HIA

However, two limitations of HIA become apparent. The first can be seen in the nature of intersectoral decision-making and it is therefore unlikely that this limitation can be removed. Each sector has its own primary objectives.

Table 2.4 *Case studies by competent political administrative level*

Local	National	International
England: King's Cross area renovation	**Denmark**: 6-per-day programme: diet and cancer	**Austria, France, Malta, Netherlands, Sweden, Switzerland:** Transport-related health effects in a transnational project
Finland: Land-use planning for a proposed residential area	**Hungary**: Obstacle-free environment for the disabled	
Italy: Wet zone creation	**Slovenia**: Common Agriculture Policy	
Lithuania: Impacts of the Klaipeda National Seaport	**Sweden**: Reconstruction of Route 73	
Netherlands: Restructuring an industrial area into a residential area	**Switzerland**: Air pollution exposure across the Alps	
Northern Ireland: City Council's Air Quality Action Plan	**Germany**: BBI Airport construction	
Poland: Erection of mobile phone base station antenna		
Republic of Ireland: Testing HIA methodology in the transport sector		
Spain: Workplace smoking restriction policy		
Wales: Remediation of a landfill refuse site		

For example, the objectives for transport, agriculture and environment may be to improve mobility, secure the availability of food through stabilization of food markets, and protect natural resources. Decisions made in these sectors will seek to contribute to primary rather than to secondary objectives such as health. In some cases, the primary sectoral objective and health may create a win–win situation, whereby the specific sectoral objectives and health go hand in hand or even reinforce each other. In many other cases, however, there will be trade-offs. For example, noise protection measures will increase the costs of a new bypass, but it will also protect the health of the population living near the new bypass.

The fact that none of the HIAs included in the case studies in this volume have resulted in the complete cancellation of the proposed plans shows that HIA is not intended to be a mechanism that hinders the planning and implementation of proposed projects, programmes and policies, but rather one that helps to show the implications of decisions in a clear light so that appropriate decisions can be made with regards to health. The benefits and losses of such decisions, however, may be unevenly distributed over different population groups. While holiday-makers and business people will benefit from new direct flight connections made possible by an airport extension, the residents in the vicinity of the airport will be exposed to additional noise emissions and pollution due to the increased air traffic. HIA has, in its best cases, contributed to the mitigation of negative effects. It is therefore a tool which brings about intersectoral, social and political compromises. Overall, it contributes to the consistency of decision-making.

There is, however, a second limitation to the effectiveness of HIA which may hinder the realization of its full potential. This second limitation is more likely to be amenable to changes as it is linked to the way and circumstances in which HIA is implemented and conducted. Three factors were analysed systematically by means of the case studies. Among them were the role of political, administrative and community-related inputs; the links between key processes, such as the policy cycle, the HIA stages and the community dynamics; and contextual factors.

Factors contributing to the effectiveness of HIA

The starting point for exploring the factors that influence the effectiveness of HIA is the analysis of the dimensions of effectiveness. The aim is to gain a better understanding of why a given HIA has a specific effectiveness profile. For example, an HIA that was analysed to be directly health and equity effective, but community ineffective, would need to look at the inputs, processes and context of that HIA to understand the various influences.

An example of political input can be seen in the Slovenian case study. Secretaries of state from different government departments envisaged HIA as an opportunity to react proactively to sectoral and health impacts caused by the accession of the country to the EU and the CAP. Although it was never an option to stop the accession process because of the health impacts, it provided an opportunity to react proactively to the changes by introducing a new nutritional policy, for example.

Community pressure and the capacity to deal with this played an important role in some of the case studies. The Welsh case study is one example of this. The authors of the Welsh case study argued that the HIA, the participatory elements involved, and the communication strategies were a precondition to move out of a situation of long-standing political stalemate.

The timing of an HIA in relation to the decision-making process turned out to be an important factor with regard to the effectiveness of HIA. Clearly, if the results of the HIA are delayed, which can happen quite easily, and if the research turns out to be unexpectedly difficult, it may be impossible to feed the results into the decision-making process and thus influence the decision. Sometimes, the research and the community have little chance to feed into the political process. Political processes can come to a halt and suddenly start all over again. The example of the BBI Airport in the German case study showed that initial recommendations may be changed for political reasons. But even if the results are fed into the decision-making process on time, the timing is still crucial with regard to the potential magnitude of the HIA. The example from Lithuania on the National Seaport development implied that if the HIA was conducted at a very late stage of the project development its influence may be limited. It is unlikely that the plans will be dropped or drastically altered because of substantial investment in the planning and the forging of political alliances in favour of a certain option.

Examples from Wales, England, Ireland, and the Netherlands (Case studies 9, 1, 16 and 4) showed the involvement of organizations that can support HIAs effectively. The Welsh HIA support unit, the London Health Observatory, the Institute for Public Health in Ireland and the Intersectoral Policy Office in the Netherlands played important role in developing, supporting or conducting HIAs.

Another contextual factor which was included in the analytical framework is the public health culture in a given country. Although public health culture is at first sight an elusive term, some dimensions of it can be made more concrete. The first dimension is the health concept that is accepted in the planning processes of other sectors. Some of the case studies, such as the Swedish, the Finnish or the Dutch ones, clearly included broad determinant-based concepts of health. In Sweden this was supported by the public health law which is based on the determinants of health. In other case studies, such as the one on the BBI Airport, a medical definition of health was employed. Other effects on the determinants of health were not considered. In fact, for the planning process, legal provisions did not allow these determinants to be included.

Is HIA a commonly used and institutionalized tool in Europe?

Chapters 3 and 4 of this book present the results of the mapping exercise and provide a rich and multifaceted description of the use and implementation of

HIA across Europe. These chapters cover a broad range of issues, including terminology; aims and values; equity; the use of HIA on different levels and in different sectors; timing; stages and types of HIA; governing, funding and costs of HIA; capacity building; and delivery of HIA.

This section includes a synthesis of the results, emphasizing the use of HIA by highlighting the uneven development and signs of progress and regress, and underlining incomplete institutionalization of HIA.

Uneven development, progress and regress

The first key result from the mapping exercise is that HIA is a common practice in only some countries. The mapping exercise identified 470 documented HIAs for the 19 countries involved in the research project. For 158 of the HIAs, reports were available and were included in a database for analysis. Most HIAs in this sample came from England, Finland, the Netherlands and Wales. Sweden was often referred to as a country with a high frequency of HIAs, but only a small number of HIAs were included in the database, as the national definition employed in Swedish public health policy defines a proper HIA to be both equity oriented and participatory. Not all HIAs are documented, especially in countries such as Sweden and Finland, where HIA procedures are included in regular decision-making at the local level (Berensson, 2004; Nilunger, Schäfer Elinder & Pettersson, 2003). Apart from this handful of countries, HIA is still in its infancy in Europe. It is subject to academic research or scientific pilot projects to explore the usefulness of the concept and the feasibility of its implementation in a specific national context.

It is also clear from the research that not all countries are making progress in the same direction. The Netherlands is an example which previously had a strong track record of HIA, including its implementation at national level. However, since the last general elections, capacities at national level were reduced and HIA became more confined to the local level (Varela Put et al., 2001). In contrast, other countries, such as Lithuania, have made health an important and obligatory component of their environmental HIA.

Incomplete institutionalization

The second key result from the mapping exercise is the incomplete institution-alization of HIA. The research results show that HIA can be implemented and institutionalized. Following a health systems model in broad terms, the governance function, funding and financing, resource generation and delivery have been researched. Given the uneven distribution in the use of HIA, some of the findings were rather surprising. For example, the researchers found many cases in which governments had started to endorse HIA either through policies, regulation or other means. Also noticeable was the basic capacity available in terms of experts and institutes supporting HIA. Some countries had even made efforts to establish dedicated support units for HIA. Even more interesting was that the research results from Finland and the Netherlands seem to demonstrate that it is possible to institutionalize HIA at national level. However, a sense of incompleteness was also apparent in the research. For example, resources useful for supporting HIA, such as databases on completed HIAs, were missing in most countries. Even a simple overview of all HIAs conducted so far was not available for many countries. Sustainable and adequate financing turned out to be a particularly difficult issue. Very few countries had made considerable provisions for financing HIAs, and even if HIA was institutionalized effectively on one level, financing was missing on the others. Incomplete institutionalization is a particular challenge to the overall effectiveness of HIA in any country. It may lead to a difficult situation if HIA activities at local level have to deal with the consequences of national policies that have not adequately taken into account health considerations.

The way forward

Based on a synthesis of the concepts, results and methodologies, the following section makes suggestions with regard to the future development of HIA. These suggestions have to be considered with great care, as the research presented in this volume has some methodological limitations, as mentioned earlier. The results of the effectiveness analysis and the mapping exercise should not be overgeneralized; indeed, the national level was researched comprehensively, while only one reference region and one reference locality were included per country. Nevertheless, the evidence seems to be conclusive enough to make five tentative suggestions.

The first suggestion is to review expectations related to HIA and adjust them according to the scientific evidence. Originally, the Gothenburg consensus, which is in many countries still a very important conceptual basis for HIA, suggests that the purpose of HIA is to promote better health for the population. In addition, four values are put forward that are believed to be particularly important to health. These are: democracy; equity; sustainable development in terms of short- and long-term perspectives, including direct and indirect effects; and the ethical use of evidence (European Centre for Health Policy, 1999 (cit. Diwan et al., 2001)). In contrast to these ambitious aims, the research presented in this volume was based on the assumption that HIA is a decision-support tool. As such it will have certain limitations, since decision-makers need to balance health objectives with the primary objectives of the pending decision, based on the sector concerned. Unless there is a win–win situation between health and the objectives of the pending decision, the HIA will always result in a compromise. Therefore, the other sector's values and objectives have to be taken into account seriously when conducting an HIA. This assumption has been supported by the case studies included in this volume. Evidence shows that these compromises are beneficial for health, although the magnitude of the influence of HIA on the pending decision varies considerably. In this regard, putting the health of the population above other aims may be an ambitious, if not untenable, aim.

The second suggestion, based on this research, is to better present the value of HIA to decision-makers in other sectors in order to strengthen its acceptance and development and to demystify some common assumptions surrounding HIA. Decision-makers in other sectors may be hesitant to integrate HIA in their decision-making processes, since it is often assumed to be "another assessment" that is costly and may eventually delay decisions and projects. The evidence presented in this book is somewhat different. It has been demonstrated that health can be integrated into other already existing assessments, as the Finnish case study has shown. It has also been shown, by the Swedish and the Welsh case studies, that HIA contributed effectively to being able to move out of impasses in the decision-making process and therefore to speeding up the process instead of delaying it. Furthermore, analysis of the different dimensions of effectiveness has provided evidence that HIA can contribute to fields beyond health. It has been beneficial for communities, administration and companies. In some of the case studies, authors argued that the HIA was a good investment since it resolved a conflict or a stalemate that was paralysing the decision-making process. The HIA avoided further delays which would have generated additional costs to the project development, as demonstrated by the Swedish case study on the reconstruction of Route 73 (Case study 8) and the Welsh case study on the remediation of a landfill refuse site (Case study 9). These are the assets of HIA that should be promoted in other sectors to complement the argument that HIA is effective with regard to equity.

The third suggestion relates to the introduction of HIA in other countries. Countries can begin using elements of HIA as a first step towards full HIA development. As argued in this volume, HIA seems to be a universal tool that can be in principle implemented successfully at all levels and linked to all sectors. This conclusion was drawn on the basis of the mapping exercise and the effectiveness analysis. Despite the universal character of HIA, HIA development across Europe varies greatly. Some countries have made great progress developing and partially institutionalizing HIA, while other countries have very little experience. Activities which use elements of HIA have purposely been included in this book. Some of them were conducted in order to explore the value of the tool for decision-making in that particular country or region. These case studies seem to have strengthened the case for HIA and demonstrated its value. In this regard, they have contributed to changing the context, paving the way for future activities even if they have not had any influence on a specific pending decision.

In addition, the case studies presented here also highlighted several important factors that contribute to effectiveness when implementing and conducting HIA:

- using specific challenges as an opportunity to implement and test HIA, as demonstrated by the Slovenian case study that covers the HIA on the effects of implementing the CAP in the course of accession to the EU;

- political leadership;

- public support;

- including health considerations at an early stage of the development – this seemed to have an advantage over those carried out at a later stage, in terms of having more of an impact on the pending decision;

- providing legal backup for the use of health determinants in the assessment – this helped to influence the decision-making process, rather than relying on a narrow medical concept of health alone;

- integrating HIA into health systems by setting up support units that can assist with concepts, methodologies and evidence; and

- clarifying who bears the cost of an HIA and, if needed, providing funding.

The fourth suggestion is that further improvement should be envisaged with regard to the quality of certain aspects of HIA. According to the case studies presented in this volume, two issues seem to be of great importance. First, the quality of communication between the various parties involved in an HIA seems to matter. This issue has been prominent in various case studies. In many of them, the potential impacts resulting from the pending decision seem to be communicated in a way that allowed for a constructive dialogue between HIA practitioners, decision-makers, stakeholders and the public. In fact, the Italian and the Welsh case studies may serve as examples where communication was proactively planned as a key aspect of the HIA. The case study on the planned erection of a mobile phone base antenna in Poland, however, has shown that such a constructive dialogue can not be taken for granted. In this case, the communication between HIA practitioners, developers, the administration and the community failed. It was therefore shown that HIAs dealing with different expectations and anxieties benefited from lessons learnt from previously completed HIAs.

Another issue which related to the quality of certain aspects of HIA was the prediction made by the HIA. However, even if the quality aspect was not part of the conceptual framework of the project, the case study on the BBI Airport planning has shown that methodologies and standards required careful review and development. In this case study, the first expert report was challenged by a second expert report and the court required a third expert report to gain a better picture which would allow them to make a legal decision. Scientific work always needs to be open to criticism, and variations in the quality cannot be ruled out. Still, it would be better to develop clearer standards on the quality of the assessment and the prediction. The currently evolving scientific discussion on the quality of the prediction is therefore a welcome contribution.

The fifth suggestion relates to the need to further link the various decision-making levels. As shown in the mapping exercise, HIA is currently strong at the local level. However, many important decisions affecting the health of the population are also made at other levels, including those made at European and international levels (by the EU, for example, and other international bodies such as the World Trade Organization (WTO)). With regard to the former, the European Commission (EC) has implemented an impact assessment capturing social, economic and environmental aspects. Health and health services are among the dimensions against which the impacts of major EU proposals are measured. A dialogue on implementation and the exchange of experiences between HIA researchers, decision-makers and practitioners would certainly contribute to the further strengthening of the practice and theory of HIA in Europe.

Many of the issues addressed in this book should not be seen in isolation from other tools and instruments of intersectoral decision- and policy-making. The work of interdepartmental committees, intersectoral health councils, interministerial working groups for developing legislation, to name just a few, is facing similar opportunities and challenges when integrating health in all policies and decisions (Sihto, Ollia & Koivusalo, 2006). It is hoped that this study provides additional insights for the development and effectiveness of these activities.

REFERENCES

Bankauskaite V, Dubois H, Saltman R (2007). Patterns of decentralization across European health systems. In: Saltman R, Bankauskaite V, Vrangbaek K, eds. *Decentralization in health care: strategies and outcomes*. Buckingham, Open University Press/McGraw Hill:22–43.

Berensson K (2004). HIA at the local level in Sweden. In: Kemm J, Parry J, Palmer S, eds. *Health impact assessment*. Oxford, Oxford University Press:213–222.

Busse R, Riesberg A (2004). *Health care systems in transition: Germany*. Copenhagen, WHO Regional Office for Europe on behalf of the European Observatory on Health Systems and Policies.

Elliott E, Williams G (2004). Developing a civic intelligence: local involvement in HIA. *Environmental Impact Assessment Review*, 24(2):231–243.

Elliott E, Williams G, Rolfe B (2004). The role of lay knowledge in HIA. In: Kemm J, Parry J, Palmer S, eds. *Health impact assessment*. Oxford, Oxford University Press:81–90.

European Centre for Health Policy (1999). Health impact assessment: main concepts and suggested approach. Gothenburg consensus paper, December 1999. In: Diwan V, et al. (2001). *Health impact assessment: from theory to practice*. Gothenburg, Nordic School of Public Health: 89–103.

Kemm J, Parry J (2004). What is HIA? Introduction and overview. In: Kemm J, Parry J, Palmer S, eds. *Health impact assessment*. Oxford, Oxford University Press:1–13.

Lock K, et al. (2004). Conducting an HIA of the effect of accession to the European Union on national agriculture and food policy in Slovenia. *Environmental Impact Assessment Review*, 24(2):177–188.

Mackenbach JP, et al. (2004). Health inequalities and HIA. In: Kemm J, Parry J, Palmer S, eds. *Health impact assessment*. Oxford, Oxford University Press:25–37.

Nilunger L, Schäfer Elinder L, Pettersson B (2003). Health impact assessment: screening of Swedish governmental inquiries. *Eurohealth*, 8(5):30–33.

Sihto M, Ollia E, Koivusalo M (2006). Principles and challenges of health in all policies. In: Ståhl T, Wismar M, Ollia E, Lahtinen E, Leppo K, eds. *Health in all policies*. Helsinki, Ministry of Social Affairs and Health:3–20.

Varela Put G, et al. (2001). *Experience with HIA at national policy level in the Netherlands. A case study*. Copenhagen, WHO Regional Office for Europe.

Wismar M (2005). The effectiveness of health impact assessment. *Eurohealth*, 10(3/4):41–43.

Wright J, Parry J, Mathers J (2005). Participation in health impact assessment: objectives, methods and core values. *Bulletin of the World Health Organization*, 83(1):58–63.

Part II
The European Map of Health Impact Assessment

Chapter 3

The use of HIA across Europe[1]

Julia Blau, Kelly Ernst, Matthias Wismar, Franz Baro,
Mojca Gabrijelčič Blenkuš, Konrade von Bremen, Rainer Fehr, Gabriel Gulis,
Tapani Kauppinen, Odile Mekel, Kirsi Nelimarkka, Kerttu Perttilä,
Nina Scagnetti, Martin Sprenger, Ingrid Stegeman and Rudolf Welteke[2]

Introduction

What do we actually know about the use of health impact assessment (HIA) in Europe? Much of the current literature is based on conceptual frameworks and case studies, or focuses on selected aspects of HIA. Most publications in the international literature refer to a limited number of countries. There is a lack of cross-country comparison applying a common conceptual and methodological framework. If HIA is discussed as a decision-making support tool and, in general, for health promotion in Europe, then it is necessary to gain a better understanding on the actual use of HIA across Europe. There might be substantial variations in the use of HIA given the differences between European countries in terms of political, socioeconomic and institutional settings.

Key questions addressed in this chapter are the following:

- How frequently is HIA used in Europe and are there variations between countries?

- Are HIA terminology and definitions uniform throughout Europe?

- Are HIA policy documents driven by the same aims and values?

---

[1] This chapter is adapted from Chapter 11 of Ståhl et al. (2006).
[2] Secondary contributors to this chapter are listed at the end of the chapter.

- Does HIA, when implemented, incorporate equity and participation?
- At what levels are HIAs implemented?
- In what sectors are HIAs found to be utilized?
- Is HIA prospective in practice?
- What are the stages and types utilized in HIA?

This chapter presents the results of a mapping exercise on the use of HIA in European countries. It can be read in conjunction with Chapter 4 (on the implementation and institutionalization of HIA in Europe) as both draw on the same data and are complementary. While this chapter focuses on the use of HIA, Chapter 4 analyses selected aspects of stewardship, funding, capacity building and HIA delivery in a comparative manner.

Since the mapping exercise presented here provides an overview on the use of HIA in Europe, conclusions on the effectiveness or quality of the HIA cannot be drawn. Parts III, IV and V of this book contain case studies that point to various dimensions of effectiveness of HIA.

The chapter is divided into seven sections. The first gives a brief overview on the conceptual framework, methodologies, limitations of the research as previously described in Chapter 2, and an overview of the data. The second compares the use of HIA definitions and terminologies across Europe. The third points to differences in the aims and values of HIA in the policy documents. The fourth explores the issues of equity and participation in practice. The fifth provides an overview of the settings of HIA by focusing on the use of HIA at different levels and in different sectors. The sixth deals with three key elements of HIA. It focuses on the timing of HIA, the stages (screening, scoping, assessing, reporting and evaluating) and the types of HIA used across Europe. Finally, a discussion draws together the different aspects of the mapping exercise.

Mapping the use of HIA in Europe

As explained in Chapter 2, the research was conceptualized as an explorative mapping exercise. The key question was: how is HIA utilized in Europe?

The conceptual framework included research both at the national and the subnational levels from 21 national entities,[3] since three of the four constituent parts of the United Kingdom (England, Scotland and Wales) were

---

[3] Austria, Belgium, Denmark, Finland, Germany, Hungary, Ireland, Italy, Lithuania, Malta, the Netherlands, Poland, Portugal, Slovakia, Slovenia, Spain, Sweden, Switzerland and the United Kingdom (denoting Wales and England; Northern Ireland is covered by the Irish contribution).

considered as national entities. Indeed, health is among the devolved competencies. Only England does not have a devolved Parliament and its health policy is determined by the United Kingdom Parliament.[4]

The conceptual framework was made operational by domestic literature research facilitated by a semi-standardized questionnaire and search strategy.

Although this research has rigorously applied conceptual frameworks and methodologies, various limitations have to be addressed especially with regard to the representativeness of the results.

1. The inclusion of an HIA was based on the dominant domestic definition of HIA. These differences in domestic definitions may result in variations with respect to the types of HIA included.

2. Excluded from the research were informal prospective assessments of possible health consequences and other forms of impact assessment if they did not embody a particularly strong health component.

3. Owing to the large number of HIAs found in England and the Netherlands, only a sample of HIAs were included.

4. Only one reference region and reference locality were selected at subnational level.

5. Two research teams did not report on any individual HIAs in their countries.

6. Some HIAs may not have been identified if they were fully integrated in the routines of an administrative structure.

Apart from all these limitations, it should be noted that this mapping exercise is the most current and the most comprehensive. A previous mapping exercise, covering 22 European countries in 2001, reported 42 HIAs either completed or in progress (EuroHealthNet, 2003).

Given the limitations mentioned above, it is impossible to determine the number of HIAs conducted in the countries. The research teams have abstracted 158 HIAs for analysis. However, adding the number of HIAs not abstracted for England and the Netherlands and the numbers provided in some domestic overviews, the overall number of documented HIAs for the countries included in the research is 470. In any case, the actual number of existing HIAs is probably much higher than the number of documented HIAs, as overviews on HIA activities were only available for nine countries.

---

[4] The Northern Ireland Assembly was suspended from October 2002 to May 2007.

Table 3.1 *HIAs as reported in the fact sheets*[a]

	1994	1995	1996	1997	1998	1999	2000	2001	2002	2003	2004	2005[b]	On-going	Yr n/a	Total
Austria						2								3	5
Belgium								1			1	1			3
Denmark									1	1					2
England					1		3	7	5	4	4	1		3	28
Finland		1		2	2	2	5	3	3	11	5				34
Germany		1		2						1	2	1			7
Hungary															0
Ireland											3				3
Italy										2	2				4
Lithuania											1				1
Malta													1		1
Netherlands			2	4	3	6	1	1	1						18
N. Ireland										2	3				5
Poland						1									1
Portugal															0
Slovakia									1						1
Slovenia	2			1	1					1	1				6
Spain								1		5		1			7
Sweden										1	4				5
Switzerland													1	2	3
Wales				1		2	5	4	3	3	6				24
Total	**2**	**2**	**2**	**10**	**7**	**13**	**14**	**17**	**16**	**29**	**32**	**6**	**3**	**5**	**158**

[a] Only HIAs reported in the fact sheets corresponding to the study were recorded in the table.

[b] The mapping exercise was completed in 2005. All HIAs completed by this time were included in 2005 and those still in progress were included under "ongoing".

Table 3.1 shows that England, Wales, Finland and the Netherlands have the highest number of HIAs reported.[5]

The results reported in Table 3.1 look surprising in regard to HIA development in Sweden especially since it has been reported that HIA has been widely employed at regional, and especially at local, level (Nilunger, Schäfer Elinder & Pettersson, 2003).

The low number of HIAs found in Sweden in the context of this study may be attributed to the fact that while gender and equity are included within the strict definition of HIA in the Swedish public health policy, HIAs that are part of an environmental impact assessment (EIA) are not included and were not reported. Therefore many EIAs, including one with a health component

---

[5] As mentioned earlier, the number of HIAs in England and the Netherlands is higher than presented in Table 3.1.

conducted by the Swedish Road Administration and other public authorities, were not incorporated in the research.

Common use of HIA definitions and terminology across Europe

A widely used definition, the so-called "Gothenburg consensus", describes HIA as "any combination of procedures or methods by which a proposed policy or programme may be judged as to the effects it may have on the health of a population" (European Centre for Health Policy, 1999 (cit. Diwan et al., 2001). There are many other definitions of HIA (Kemm and Parry, 2004; Krieger et al., 2003). Still, most researchers would agree on two central features of HIA as argued by John Kemm in Chapter 1.

- It attempts to predict the health consequences of different options.

- It is intended to influence and assist decision-makers.

According to the data collected, the Gothenburg consensus still provides a general framework of orientation for HIA according to the analysis of policy documents, legal acts and other key supportive documents for many countries. In seven countries, the Gothenburg consensus plays an explicit role in the description or definition of HIA.

The use of the English term "health impact assessment" is widespread; it is used in 16 countries. Among these countries, 11 also translate the term into the national language. The remaining five countries use the term exclusively in their own language. However, as the German and Swiss case study shows (see Box 3.1), translations may have strategic connotations, and these connotations may have consequences on the use of HIA. Additionally, the Danish case study (see Box 3.2) provides an example of a translation that may cover activities not considered as HIA in other countries.

Differences in aims and values of HIA in the documents

While there is a great deal of uniformity in the use and definitions of HIA, there are marked differences in the aims and values. The influential Merseyside Guidelines have strongly emphasized the case for explicit values and equity (Scott-Samuel, Birley & Ardern, 1998).

The aims of public policy dictate that HIA should openly declare its values and that social, material and environmental equity should feature strongly among them. This is because public policy impacts disproportionately on the already disadvantaged. Consistent with the adoption of an equity-focused

Box 3.1 *Case study of the terminology and definition of HIA in Germany and Switzerland*

In German, *Gesundheitsverträglichkeitsprüfung* (GVP) is often used for the translation of HIA and roughly means "examination of acceptability from a health perspective". The term was created in analogy to *Umweltverträglichkeitsprüfung* (UVP). UVP is a widely accepted and officially used translation of EIA, which is a legal obligation in the Member States of the European Union. The analogy was strategically intended to suggest that GVP is similar to or part of UVP and therefore holds comparable importance and legal implications. It is clear that both German terms are far from being "literal" translations, and the term GVP met with much criticism. First, it evokes bureaucratic and "red-tape" associations. Second, sometimes the very existence of GVP is questioned since there is no legal basis. Still others claim that nearly every UVP already constitutes a GVP, simply because it considers noise and pollution levels relevant to human health. In short, GVP is a problematic term. Therefore, in the scientific debate, one often uses the English term HIA. In practical applications, a variety of alternative terms exist, for example *Mitwirkung in Planung*, which looks at the entire planning process but has a more legal and administrative context. Switzerland has adopted the German GVP for its German-speaking regions. It is considered as a translation of HIA, despite the fact that HIA is translated into the three regional languages.

Box 3.2 *Case study of the terminology and definition of HIA in Denmark*

In Denmark, the definition of HIA often comes from the Gothenburg consensus paper and is translated into Danish. The official translation is *sundhedskonsekvensvurdering*. In addition, the term *sundhedsmaessige konsekvenser*, which means health-related consequences, is often used. However, it tends to be applied more in relation to economic evaluation. The term "health impact assessment" can be found in literature and database searches that focus more on economic and environmental areas than on health. The terminology restricts the scope of HIA and therefore the broader social determinants of health are not addressed.

approach are the use of participatory methods which fully involve those affected by the public policy at every stage of assessment, and the openness of all stages of the HIA process to public scrutiny.

The Gothenburg consensus stresses the importance of values as well, focusing on democracy, equity, sustainable development and ethical use of evidence.

For the analysis of aims and values, a synopsis of five objectives was drawn from the literature (Kemm & Parry, 2004; Mindell, Ison & Joffe, 2003) as presented in the row headings of Table 3.2. However, not all countries,

Table 3.2 *The objectives of HIA as reported in the analysed sample of documents*

	National level	Reference region	Reference locality
Countries with relevant documents included in the analysis	16	8	11
Objectives in documents			
To maximize health gain or minimize loss	9	3	6
To tackle health inequalities and inequities	8	4	3
To raise awareness among decision-makers of the relationship between health and the physical, social and economic environment, thereby ensuring that they always include a consideration of health consequences in their deliberations	11	6	8
To help decision-makers identify and assess possible health consequences and optimize overall outcome of a decision	12	6	4
To help those affected by policies to participate in policy formulation and contribute to decision-making	5	2	2

reference regions and reference localities have relevant documents such as governmental policies, strategy documents or delivery plans, so it was not always possible to identify the objectives of HIA in a given country. Also, in some countries, the regional and/or the local level are not concerned with decision-making, while in other countries decision-making bodies exist at all three levels.

The small number of documents available makes it difficult to provide numerical comparisons of objectives. However, it can be seen from the available data that objectives that related to the decision-makers (to raise awareness among decision-makers and to help decision-makers) ranked particularly high at all levels. This is important as it stresses the objective of HIA to influence the decision-making process. However, other objectives such as equity and participation are less frequently mentioned.

The practice of HIA values

Equity and participation are issues that have attracted a great deal of attention in the debate on HIA. In the policy documents, regulations and other supporting documents analysed, equity and participation ranked surprisingly low. The purpose of the analysis of the individual 158 HIAs was to clarify the role of equity and participation in the practice of HIA.

Table 3.3 *Factors to stratify HIA in order to take health inequalities into account*

	Stratified by conventional factors	Stratified by specific factors
National level	4	24
Reference region	6	9
Reference locality	17	17

Equity

Equity is a highly debated issue in the literature on HIA. However, the analysis of objectives of HIA has revealed that not all policy documents, regulations and other HIA documents place equity equally high on the agenda. It has been argued that analysing the distribution of health impacts over various groups is a complex, scientifically demanding and time- and resource-consuming task. It is assumed that the equity claim often falls short in the execution of HIA.

In contrast to the analysis of the objectives of HIA, most of the HIAs identified by the project had an equity concern. The identified 158 HIAs were analysed to see if they were stratified by group in order to take inequalities into account. Stratifying the population is a condition for assessing the distribution of health impacts over a given population. Conventional factors for stratification are, for example, gender, age and socioeconomic group. However, specific interventions may require specific stratification. A policy that may increase exposure to pollution may have severe health impacts for those who already suffer from a respiratory condition, while the health impact for others may be negligible. A total of 71 HIAs reported the stratification of the population either into conventional or special categories highlighting the general concern for equity. In six cases, both conventional and special categories were employed (see Table 3.3).

The Welsh case study (see Box 3.3) provides an example of a health inequality impact assessment (HIIA).

Participation

Participation is also a highly debated issue in HIA and one that can be addressed from different angles. There is a strong emphasis on democracy as a value in itself. Whenever possible, citizens should have a say in the decision. From a more technical point of view, it is argued that the affected population is an important source of information. Learning about the concerns of the affected population and stakeholders may help to get a better understanding of the consequences of the pending decision. This is especially helpful in

Box 3.3 *Case study of health inequality impact assessment (HIIA) in a road construction project in Wales*

Reducing health inequalities is one of the priorities of the Welsh Assembly Government. HIAs that focus on the health equity impact of specific measures are an important way of achieving this. An HIA was applied to analyse the impact of a road construction project that would link the motorway between Cardiff and London. The road would be located very close to a housing area that consisted primarily of rental units, leased out on the basis of social criteria. The area suffered from high levels of unemployment and very low incomes. A rapid HIA, initiated by the local residents' association, was carried out, using the Bro Taf method. This was devised in the former Bro Taf health authority area of Wales, and has been somewhat expanded and revised to become a useful source of information alongside Wales's national guidance on HIA (WHIASU, 2004). One of the main tasks of the HIA was to discuss and document health impacts on the already vulnerable. The HIA took into account issues such as the health impacts of pollution, noise and physical activity levels. The evidence collected led to the conclusion that the road construction project would have negative health impacts on the local population. The outcome of the HIA was positive in that it empowered a vulnerable group to raise their concerns, while making planners aware of the impact of their activities. The road has not been built, although it is uncertain to what extent the results of the HIA influenced this decision (Fosse, 2005; Lester & Temple, 2004).

identifying vulnerable groups in the affected population and assessing the distribution of impacts on the population. A third approach discusses the value of community development. The involvement of stakeholders and the affected community has positive secondary effects. Strengthening communities by including them in the decision-making process may raise awareness of health issues and strengthen the community's capacity to tackle these issues. Related to this is the assumed capability of participation in an HIA that may help to resolve conflicts within a given community. The project shows the majority of the HIAs reported were participatory: 102 out of 158; 29 were not participatory and in 27 cases it was unclear, or data were insufficient to assess the participatory nature of the HIA.

While participation does not feature highly on the policy documents identified, it is indeed an important feature of HIA in practice as seen from the project data. Participation seems particularly strong at local level, as seen in Figure 3.1, where it appears that HIA at the reference localities tended to use a more participatory approach than at the national and regional levels.

In the analysis, three forms of participation were distinguished: the right to be informed, the right to be heard and the right to decide. According to the data,

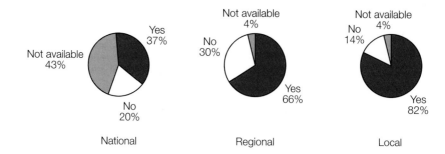

Figure 3.1 *Community and stakeholder participation in HIA as reported in the fact sheets*

the right to be informed goes hand in hand with the right to be heard. This implies a rather active involvement of stakeholders and the affected populations. In most cases, after the completion of the HIA, the report was made available to the public. In 70 cases, both rights were exerted stressing the importance of community-based involvement in strengthening the HIAs' recommendations to allow them to be tailored closely to the needs of the current population. The right to decide was identified in only 11 cases implying that this is a more difficult area to address. It is clear that participation and transparency are closely connected and the project results highlight this with 138 out of 158 HIA reports being made available to the public.

HIA settings: levels and sectors

The relevance attached to HIA is at least partly owed to its assumed capacity to be used as a universal mechanism that can be applied equally to all sectors. Case studies in the literature range from supranational (Hübel & Hedin, 2003; Mekel et al., 2004), national (Roscam Abbing, 2004) and regional to local HIAs. They deal with issues such as the common agricultural policies (Dahlgren, Nordgren & Whitehead, 1996), accession to the EU (Lock et al., 2004), extension of airports (Abdel Aziz, Radford & McCabe, 2004), urban reconstruction schemes (Bekker, Putters & van der Grinten, 2005) or the proposed burning of old tyres in a cement plant (Cook & Kemm, 2004). This raises the question: are these exceptional cases or does this reflect common practice with respect to HIAs?

Levels

Among the 158 HIAs included in the mapping exercise, 54 were conducted at national level, 23 at regional level and 81 at local level. While the results need to be carefully interpreted in the context of the methodologies employed, it

Box 3.4   *Case study of national and regional levels of HIA in Slovenia*

Slovenia has a long tradition of assessing impacts on health. Procedures are, however, embedded in the legislation and are only partially comparable with HIA methodology. The Ministry of Health of Slovenia has started to implement HIA as a method at national level. A model of HIA on food and agricultural policies related to accession to the EU has been developed. The process resulted in better cooperation between the agricultural and health sectors. The outcome of this cooperation was the inclusion of the food security pillar as an important part of the resolution on the national food and nutrition action plan. Similar to the national level, comparable procedures for assessing impacts on health have been used at regional level, where Slovenia came the closest to HIA in the area of environmental issues. In some regions, long-term measures were put in place to assess the impact of environmental policies such as waste management, air pollution and drinking water management. In these cases, efforts to reduce environmentally related harm were at the forefront of the country's attention with the aim of preventing direct negative impacts on the health of the exposed population. In these activities, regional development agencies with their intersectoral potential have been recognized as an important partner for future structural capacity building in support of HIA.

was expected that at national level HIA would be more prominent, as this level was searched comprehensively. Since only one reference region and one reference locality were selected per country, it is not possible to extrapolate this information within countries and/or between countries. However, it is interesting to note that more HIAs were taking place at these levels. There are differences in institutional settings in some countries, where decision-making and HIA only take place at two levels, meaning that in addition to the national level, HIA is only taking place either at regional or local level, as the Slovenian case study shows (see Box 3.4).

In general, the data obtained from the analysis of the 158 HIAs suggest that while HIAs are taking place at all levels, HIAs at national level are rather scarce. There could be a variety of reasons for this, including the possibility of a lack of support for HIA at national level or the fact that many countries are still in the infancy stages of implementing HIA.

Sectors

Health impact assessment is viewed as a key mechanism for intersectoral health. Does HIA keep its intersectoral promise? Is it really applicable to a large variety of sectors? From the project data, HIA is found to be fulfilling its intersectoral promise and is conducted in a variety of sectors. Overall, HIA is most commonly found in the transport, housing and urban planning,

Table 3.4 *Sectors of HIA*

Sector	Transport	Housing/ urban planning	Environment	Multisectoral	Health	Other	Employment	Social care	Finance	Energy	Agriculture	Industry	Education	Tourism
Number of HIAs	27	23	18	17	14	10	10	8	8	7	7	4	3	2

environmental and multisectoral sectors. Most of the HIAs reported were carried out outside of the health and social sectors (see Table 3.4).

Depending on the level, some sectors are more prominent than others. At national level, the four main sectors are transport, housing, finance and health. At regional level, employment is the most common sector, followed by transport, social care and environment.[6] At local level, housing is the most common sector, followed by multisectoral, transport and environment. However, all these data have to be interpreted with great care owing to the small number of cases and the aforementioned methodological limitations. Still, the analysis provides evidence that it is possible to conduct HIA in a large variety of sectors.

Transport can be found at all levels, which shows that there are health concerns at all levels when transport issues are involved. The Austrian (see Box 3.5) and Belgian (see Box 3.6) case studies illustrate this.

Differences in timing, stages and types of HIA

This section reviews the timing of HIA, the use of stages (screening, scoping, assessing, reporting, evaluating) and the use of different types of assessment.

Prospective timing

There has been a long conceptual debate on the timing of HIA. While it is generally accepted that HIA is prospective, it has been argued that there may be the need for concurrent or retrospective HIA. Concurrent HIA is conducted during implementation to identify changes as they occur and allow for action to be taken. Retrospective HIA is carried out after the proposal has been implemented; this may be more of an evaluation exercise which can, in turn, influence similar future decisions. Although HIA can be defined differently in a multitude of countries, the Gothenburg consensus is seen to be

---

[6] An extended HIA is sometimes conducted in the framework of EIA.

Box 3.5 *Case study of the transport sector in Austria and five other European countries*

Austria is extensively affected by transit and transport policies and most of the HIAs
are aimed at this sector. However, the lack of consistent methods to assess the overall
health impacts of transport policies has led to a conglomeration of different concepts,
ranging from narrow mono-disciplinary expertise to comprehensive interdisciplinary
assessments. A transnational project (Austria, France, Malta, the Netherlands, Sweden
and Switzerland), coordinated by Austria, started in 2003. The aim of the project was
to provide a review on transport-related health impacts, costs and benefits and to
make a set of evidence-based recommendations on political implementation strategies
with a particular focus on children. Along with the review of the scientific literature, the
project facilitated a series of four two-day workshops in which the participants were
experts and stakeholders on health, transport, environment, economy, children's affairs,
scientists, governmental and nongovernmental representatives, and representatives
from the Organisation for Economic Co-operation and Development (OECD), United
Nations Economic Commission for Europe (UNECE) and World Health Organization
(WHO). A comprehensive brochure covers the main outcome, conclusions and
recommendations. The results were presented at the Fourth WHO Ministerial
Conference on Environment and Health in 2004.

Box 3.6 *Case study of the transport sector in Belgium: Brussels Airport*

In the area around Brussels Airport, nightly air traffic has economic advantages due
to employment. The negative health and economic impacts have not been directly
investigated. A health economics impact model was developed in order to assess the
burden related to sleep disturbance due to noise from airplanes. Data were based on
observed noise levels in the area around Brussels Airport and published relationships
between noise levels and the probability of sleep disturbance. Hence, per town or
village in the area, the incremental percentage of the population suffering from sleep
disturbance was calculated. Based on literature, a causal relationship was found
between sleep disturbance and alcohol abuse, heart disease, diabetes, depression
and overall mortality. Hence, owing to the excess in sleep disturbance, 2644 more
alcohol abuse patients, 758 more patients with heart disease, 580 more cases of
diabetes, 5492 more incidents of depression and 215 more deaths occurred in the
area. As these diseases are associated with direct medical costs and with productivity-
related costs, the total societal impact was estimated at €149 991 730. The health
impact was found to be higher than originally expected, and the negative economic
consequences of the health impact were taken into account when looking at the
positive employment effect.

widely accepted. The project results indicate that most countries do indeed conduct HIA prospectively in order to influence decision-makers. Based on the 158 fact sheets, HIA timing is predominantly prospective (65%). However, in some countries – such as Austria, Belgium, the Netherlands, Slovakia, Slovenia and Switzerland – the HIAs tend to be conducted concurrently or retrospectively. Countries that report concurrent or retrospective HIAs may see HIA as a form of evaluation rather than a tool to influence current decision-making. Alternatively, they may have planned to start – or may have started – the HIA prospectively, but owing to time constraints or other factors the project carried on and the HIA was therefore conducted concurrently or retrospectively. An example of this can be seen in an HIA conducted on traffic and transport in the Republic of Ireland. While it was intended to conduct the HIA prospectively, by the time an agreement was reached by the different stakeholders, the project had gone ahead, but it was decided it was still worth pursuing retrospectively.

Stages

According to the Gothenburg consensus, HIA is conducted in five stages. The first stage – screening – primarily filters out proposals that do not require HIA, so that scarce resources are used efficiently. Screening encompasses identifying the elements or aspects of the proposal to be assessed such as the aims and objectives of the HIA, the values underpinning the HIA, and so on. The second stage – scoping – serves to determine the methods that need to be used. The third stage – appraisal or assessment – identifies and calculates the health impacts of a proposal. The fourth stage – reporting – focuses on preparing and submitting the report with its recommendations integrating the information obtained from stakeholders during appraisal. For the submission, it is necessary for the report to be submitted within the schedule set for the relevant decision-making process. Submission of the report to decision-makers is the primary mechanism by which the outputs from appraisal influence proposal development and/or implementation. The fifth stage – monitoring and evaluation – has several components: process evaluation assesses how successful the process was in practice; impact evaluation monitors the acceptance and implementation of recommendations; and outcome evaluation monitors indicators and health outcomes after the proposal has been implemented (Mindell, Ison & Joffe, 2003).

Table 3.5 shows that scoping, appraisal and reporting are the most widely used stages of HIA. The evaluations of HIAs (both process and outcome evaluations) are minimal, most likely due to limited financial and personnel resources remaining once the HIAs are completed. Not all HIAs followed all

Table 3.5 *Stages of HIA as reported in the fact sheets*

Stage completed	Screening	Scoping	Appraisal	Reporting	Evaluation
Yes	84	102	122	138	49
No	69	51	31	13	95
Not available	5	5	5	7	14

the stages. In only 39 cases, four stages of the HIA were completed, and all five stages were completed in only 29 cases.

Types of HIA

According to the conceptual framework based on a review of key documents, three types of HIA were distinguished in the research.

The first type is a mini or desktop HIA. It can be defined as "a brief investigation of the health impacts of a proposal" and usually involves an exchange of existing knowledge and expertise, and research from previous HIAs. This process usually takes a few days to complete.

The second type is a standard or intermediate HIA. It can be defined as "a more detailed investigation of health impacts" and usually involves a review of the available evidence, exploration of opinions, experiences and expectations, and sometimes the production and analysis of new information. This more lengthy investigation can take weeks to complete.

The third type is a maxi or comprehensive HIA. It can be defined as "an intensive investigation of health impacts undertaken over an extended period" and usually involves a review of the available evidence base along with the other elements mentioned under the second type. In addition, it also involves the production and analysis of new information and may take months to complete.

In the HIAs reported (see Figure 3.2), the most commonly used type of HIA at national level and in the reference localities was the standard or intermediate (22 HIAs out of 54 at national level and 35 out of 81 at local level). At regional level, however, the mini or desktop HIA was used most frequently (13 out of 23). The full-scale HIA known as maxi or comprehensive was used less frequently than other types. This may be a result of the maxi HIA taking a considerable amount of time, and being seen as a possible drain on staff and financial resources. From the project data, Italy, England and Spain (HIAs in the sample) were the three countries that exceptionally undertook most of their HIAs as maxi or comprehensive. Not all countries are able to allocate the necessary resources for such an exercise, therefore the limitations of the HIA must be taken into account.

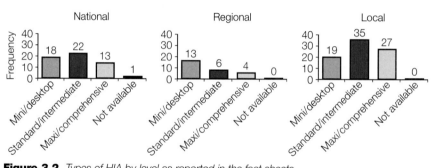

Figure 3.2 *Types of HIA by level as reported in the fact sheets*

Box 3.7 *Case study of a mini HIA at national level in Finland*

In Finland, it is a common practice that a (mini) HIA is a part of the more comprehensive assessment process EIA, strategic environmental assessment (SEA)). The assessment is also usually integrated into the preparation of the proposal and report as in this example of the "housing policy programme approved by the government for 2004–2006".
The Ministry of the Environment commissioned the assessment of the housing policy programme. It established a special working group for conducting the HIA. The Ministry consisted of experts from various sectors and institutions such as the Ministry of the Environment, Ministry of Social Affairs and Health, an association of residential property managers, etc. The working group developed both the programme and its assessment. The group functioned as an expert panel and prepared the programme in six months. An assessment expert from the Ministry of the Environment made the appraisal of economic, environmental and human impacts by himself in one day. The appraisal was discussed and approved by the working group during one meeting and they submitted the programme to the government. The working group identified impacts on regional policy as well as socio-political impacts (that is, impacts on housing of different population groups and equitable housing policy). The assessment paid attention to housing of low-income people and specific groups. The impacts on health and living conditions were also assessed.

The Finnish case study (see Box 3.7) provides an example of a mini HIA at national level.

Conclusion

The mapping exercise presented in this chapter provides an overview on the use of HIA in Europe. The data have to be interpreted with great care, especially since only one reference region and one reference locality were investigated per country. Furthermore, HIAs that are fully integrated in administrative procedures may not leave any trace in terms of a report or a publication and can therefore not be included in the analysis.

However, despite these limitations, two conclusions regarding the current use of HIA can be drawn. First, HIA has proven its capacity to be used in various countries at various levels and in various sectors. Equity and participation, two values which are widely discussed in the debate on HIA, play a substantial role in the practice of HIA. The evidence also provides insight into the timing, stages and types of HIA. Despite all the variations reported, HIA can, in principle, be used prospectively, cover all stages and use different types of HIA.

Given the long period covered by the research, it is surprising that only a few countries have used HIA extensively. This uneven development may have different reasons. In some countries, HIA development started much earlier than in others. Some have a long track record in using HIA while others are just about to develop HIA. These differences may be due to a lack of government support, funding, capacity building and establishing mechanisms for delivery. However, they may also reflect the difficulty HIA has in proving its usefulness to other sectors and to therefore become a systematic part of the policy-making process, rather than a tool that is employed on an ad hoc basis for pilot studies. In Parts III, IV and V of this book, the effectiveness of HIA on the policy-making process is analysed through country-specific case studies, at various levels of development.

But is HIA a decision-support tool for all levels? In many countries key policies are formulated at national level. Little HIA activity has been reported at national level although this level was researched comprehensively. Policy-making also takes place at subnational level. Owing to federalization, decentralization and devolution, important political accountabilities and competencies can be found at regional level. It is not possible to extrapolate the results from the reference regions to all other regions but the information provided raises some scepticism of the current use of HIA as a decision-support tool for all levels. In fact, most HIAs identified were conducted in the reference localities.

Secondary contributors to this chapter

Elisabet Aldenberg, Swedish National Institute of Public Health, Sweden; Francisco Barroso Martin, Técnicas de Salud S.A., Spain; Ceri Breeze, Welsh Assembly Government, Wales, United Kingdom; Edit Eke, Semmelweis University, Hungary; Alison Golby, Cardiff University, Wales, United Kingdom; Loes M van Herten, TNO Quality of Life, The Netherlands; Jarmila Korcova, Trnava University, Slovakia; Owen Metcalfe, The Institute of

Public Health in Ireland; Ewa Nowak, CM Jagiellonian University, Poland; José Pereira-Miguel, University of Lisbon, Portugal; Roberta Siliquini, University of Turin, Italy; Marius Stricka, Kaunas University of Medicine, Lithuania; Lorraine Taylor, former Health Development Agency, United Kingdom.

REFERENCES

European Centre for Health Policy (1999). Health impact assessment: main concepts and suggested approach. Gothenburg consensus paper, December 1999. In: Diwan V, et al., eds. *Health impact assessment: from theory to practice*. Gothenburg, Nordic School of Public Health: 89–103 (http://www.euro.who.int/ document/PAE/Gothenburgpaper.pdf, accessed 26 July 2007).

Abdel Aziz MI, Radford J, McCabe J (2004). The Finningley Airport HIA: a case study. In: Kemm J, Parry J, Palmer S, eds. *Health impact assessment*. Oxford, Oxford University Press: 285–298.

Bekker MPM, Putters K, van der Grinten TED (2005). Evaluating the impact of HIA on urban reconstruction decision-making. Who manages whose risks? *Environmental Impact Assessment Review*, 25(7–8):758–771.

Cook A, Kemm J (2004). Health impact assessment of proposal to burn tyres in a cement plant. *Environmental Impact Assessment Review*, 24(2):207–216.

Dahlgren G, Nordgren P, Whitehead M (1996). *Health impact assessment of the EU Common Agricultural Policy*. Stockholm, National Institute of Public Health.

EuroHealthNet (2003). *Health impact assessment and government policymaking in European countries: a position report*. Cardiff, Public Health Strategy Division, Office of the Chief Medical Officer, Welsh Assembly Government.

Fosse E (2005). *Social inequality in health as a theme of health impact assessments. Tools and experiences in some European countries*. (Report to the Norwegian Directorate of Health and Social Affairs.)

Hübel M, Hedin A (2003). Developing health impact assessment in the European Union. *Bulletin of the World Health Organization*, 81(6):463–464.

Kemm J, Parry J (2004). What is HIA? Introduction and overview. In: Kemm J, Parry J, Palmer S, eds. *Health impact assessment*. Oxford, Oxford University Press: 1–13.

Krieger N, et al. (2003). Assessing health impact assessment: multidisciplinary and international perspectives. *Journal of Epidemiology and Community Health*, 57:659–662.

Lester C, Temple M (2004). Rapid collaborative health impact assessment: a three-meeting process. *Public Health*, 118(3):218–224.

Lock K, et al. (2004). Conducting an HIA of the effect of accession to the European Union on national agriculture and food policy in Slovenia. *Environmental Impact Assessment Review*, 24(2):177–188.

Mekel O, et al. (2004). *Policy health impact assessment for the European Union: pilot health impact assessment of the European Employment Strategy in Germany*. Liverpool, IMPACT, University of Liverpool.

Mindell J, Ison E, Joffe M (2003). A glossary for health impact assessment. *Journal of Epidemiology and Community Health*, 57:647–651.

Nilunger L, Schäfer Elinder L, Pettersson B (2003). Health impact assessment: screening of Swedish governmental inquiries. *Eurohealth*, 8(5):30–33.

Roscam Abbing EW (2004). HIA and national policy in the Netherlands. In: Kemm J, Parry J, Palmer S, eds. *Health impact assessment*. Oxford, Oxford University Press: 177–190.

Scott-Samuel A, Birley M, Ardern K (1998). *Merseyside guidelines for health impact assessment*. Liverpool, Merseyside Health Impact Assessment Steering Group/Liverpool Public Health Observatory.

Ståhl T, et al., eds. (2006). *Health in all policies: prospects and potentials*. Helsinki, Ministry of Social Affairs and Health, 189–207.

WHIASU (2004). *Improving health and reducing health inequalities: a practical guide to health impact assessment*. Cardiff, Welsh Health Impact Assessment Support Unit, Welsh Assembly Government (http://new.wales.gov.uk/docrepos/40382/cmo/reports/pre-06/improving-health-e?lang=en, accessed 26 July 2007).

Chapter 4
Implementing and institutionalizing HIA in Europe[7]

Matthias Wismar, Julia Blau, Kelly Ernst, Eva Elliott, Alison Golby,
Loes van Herten, Teresa Lavin, Marius Strička, Gareth Williams[8]

Introduction

The purpose of this chapter is to analyse implementation and institutionaliza-tion of health impact assessment (HIA) in Europe. It will support the debate on how to advance with HIA developments in the countries concerned and how HIA can be a decision-support tool. The chapter will also raise the question as to whether institutionalization is really a tenable option for all countries included in the research, given the differences in current developments (as highlighted in Chapter 3).

The debate on implementation has centred on the issue of institutionalizing HIA. Institutionalizing is a multifaceted concept defined in various ways by disciplines such as sociology, political sciences and organizational theory (Banken, 2001). In the context of the debate on HIA, institutionalizing means the systematic integration of HIA into the decision-making process. HIA would have to become part of the rules and procedures normally followed by the different decision-making bodies involved in order to realize its potential to catalyse intersectoral action for health (Banken, 2003).

Institutionalization as an approach is not unchallenged. It has been argued that it may restrict the scope for political advocacy since it requires an impartial role of the HIA practitioner. It has also been stressed that, prior to institutionalization, methodological standardization is required. However,

[7] This chapter is adapted from Chapter 12 of Ståhl et al. (2006).
[8] Secondary contributors to this chapter are listed at the end of the chapter.

many methodological issues are still the subject of scientific debate. Among these are the quality of prediction, the quantification of impacts, the analysis of distribution of impacts over a given population, the role of the practitioner and participation (Kemm, 2005a; 2005b). Moreover, it has been stressed that each country will need to find its own approach to institutionalizing HIA according to the specific domestic contextual circumstances (Banken, 2003). While these arguments are all valid, institutionalization remains an important if not key perspective for HIA. First, if conducted on an ad hoc basis there is the danger of opportunistic HIAs. HIAs may only be initialized if the outcome is expected to support a preferred policy decision. This reduces the potential of HIA substantially. Second, it is doubtful if criteria-based priorities can be addressed by HIAs conducted on an ad hoc basis. Even the undertaking of a large number of HIAs in a given country does not necessarily mean that those policies and decisions, which matter most in terms of health consequences and should therefore be prioritized, are subject to an HIA. Third, if not institutionalized, HIAs will depend on proactive political leadership, administration and communities, but these circumstances cannot be expected everywhere. Fourth, if not institutionalized, positive developments may become easily subject to political volatilities and be reversed quickly. Fifth – and this is probably the experience many HIA practitioners can relate to – if not institutionalized there is little leverage for the results of the HIA predicting serious negative health consequences of a pending decision being taken into consideration by the decision-makers. All of this does not mean that HIAs conducted on an ad hoc basis have no value. The point is that ad hoc HIAs have their limits.

The key message of the chapter is that it is possible to institutionalize HIA. There is evidence that some countries have at least partially institutionalized HIA. However, despite these promising examples, it remains doubtful if insti-tutionalization of HIA is currently an option for all countries. Institutionalization requires firm political commitment and strong stewardship. It also requires investment into HIA and resource generation. Institutionalization does not come about without effort and does require constant support. It should also be taken into consideration that some countries have a stronger public health culture and capacity in support of insti-tutionalization than others.

Summing up the evidence presented later in this chapter, HIA implementation and institutionalization are incomplete in all countries. None of the countries have strengthened and developed all the stewardship, funding, resource generation and delivery in full. This is an important limiting factor for HIA activities. The variations in implementing HIA explain the uneven distribution of HIA activities across Europe. However, despite the incompleteness, there is evidence that some countries have made progress in implementing and institutionalizing HIA. Stewardship for HIA has been strengthened in many countries by national, regional and local governments. However, HIA is not always endorsed at subnational levels. In some cases, policy has not resulted in regulation and in other cases, regulation seems to come without vision and policy. Apart from some notable exceptions, the provision of HIA-related basic health intelligence is currently underdeveloped. Financing remains a key issue and limiting factor to the implementation of HIA. So far, only a handful of countries have invested in HIA in terms of securing and providing dedicated and substantial budgets both for generating resources and conducting HIA. Moreover, solid information on the costs of different types of HIA is still scarce. Resource generation and capacity building are supported by a multitude of organizations and institutions. In some cases, there is evidence of complementary or coordinated activities. According to the data from the sample, the delivery of HIA is relatively strongly developed. The evidence shows that most countries have established "lead agencies" which can act as focal points exerting technical leadership and providing support regarding conducting, organizing, managing, commissioning and supervising the HIA. For the choice of assessors, a multitude of different options were reported. These options, depending on the type and topic of HIA, include administrators, state institutes, universities, private research companies and freelance scientists. Some countries have managed to establish a close link between the pending decision and the triggering of the HIA process. However, in most countries, this link is less solidly institutionalized and makes HIA dependent on proactive initiatives. Similar to the link between a pending decision and triggering the HIA process, some countries have managed to establish a close link between the assessment and the reporting of the HIA to the decision-makers.

This introduction is followed by a brief mention of the data and methodology and a section on comparing HIA implementation and institutionalization. The results are presented in four subsections on selected aspects of stewardship, funding, capacity building and delivery of HIA. Finally, the results will be discussed in regard to HIA as a tool to support decision-making and further developments of HIA.

Data and methodology

The results and analysis presented in this chapter are based on an explorative mapping exercise conducted in 2005. The methodology and limitations are explained in Chapter 2. To avoid misunderstandings, three limitations in regard to the representativeness of the results have to be highlighted.

1. The inclusion of an HIA was based on the dominant domestic definition of HIA. These differences in domestic definitions may result in variations with respect to the types of HIA included.

2. Only one reference region and reference locality were selected at subnational level.

3. Not all countries have completed the questionnaire at all levels.

Comparing implementation and institutionalization of HIA

There is currently no established conceptual framework for analysing implementation and institutionalization of HIA. In order to facilitate analysis and comparison, this chapter draws on concepts developed in health systems research (WHO, 2000). In health systems research, it is assumed that systems work to achieve specific goals such as the health of the population, the nonmedical expectations of patients and citizens or the fair distribution of the financial burden of health systems expenditure. Achievement of these goals will depend on the development of four functions. These four functions are: stewardship, sometimes used interchangeably with good governance; financing; resource generation; and delivery. These functions can be subdivided into many detailed tasks. The research has focused on a selection of key tasks and aspects of these functions, while some of the case studies presented in the chapter provide a broader picture on the functions.

One of the reasons for using this conceptual framework is the degree of abstraction. It allows comparison between diverse forms of implementation and institutionalization. This is important given the institutional, social and economic diversity of Europe. It is also important to use abstract categories for the analytical framework to avoid imposing strict definitions of HIA. This would not allow for identifying and analysing the assumed diversity of institutionalizing and implementing HIA.

Selected aspects of stewardship for HIA

Stewardship is a function which is primarily, but not exclusively, conducted by the government. In broad terms, it is concerned with the welfare of the population. In this regard, stewardship shall provide the framework, support and supervision towards the development of a decision-support tool. Stewardship can be divided into three tasks: policy formulation (vision, values,

Table 4.1 *Policy, regulation or other means of endorsement to provide a framework and basis for action for HIA*

	Austria	Belgium	Denmark	England	Finland	Germany	Hungary	Ireland	Italy	Lithuania	Malta	Netherlands	Northern Ireland	Poland	Portugal	Slovakia	Slovenia	Spain	Sweden	Switzerland	Wales
National	O	O		P	P	O	P	O			O	R	O	P	R	O	P	R		P		P
Reference region		R	O	O		R								R		R			P	R	
Reference locality	P	P		R					O	O		R	O	R	P				P		O

P, policy; R, regulation; O, other means of endorsement.

policies, evaluation, etc.), exerting influence (promoting the issue, paralleling political processes, involving stakeholders, consensus building, setting incentives and sanctions, etc.) and gathering and providing health intelligence (WHO, 2000; Saltman & Ferrousier-Davis, 2000; Travis et al., 2003). The following two subsections focus on selected aspects of stewardship. In the first subsection, the existence of policies, regulations and other means of endorsement for HIA are reviewed. This is followed by a second subsection which provides an overview on selected aspects of health intelligence for HIA.

Policies, regulations and other means of endorsement

To understand how governments and ministries fulfil their stewardship roles, an analysis of the means of HIA endorsement was conducted. Do governments support the development of HIA by some kind of official document and if so are they employing policies, regulations[9] or other means of endorsement in order to provide a framework and basis for action for HIA?

As presented in Table 4.1, almost all of the countries included in the research had at least a policy, regulation or other means of endorsement either at national level or at the level of the reference region or reference locality.

A well-known example of a policy that includes HIA is *Saving lives: our healthier nation* (Secretary of State for Health, 1999), policy in England from 1999. This policy has been superseded by a more recent public health policy, which is suggesting that non-health sector impacts on health should be more routinely considered before implementation through HIA, for example. However, detailed provisions have not been made (Department of Health, 2004). In Wales, HIA has been in policy documents since 1998 (see Box 4.1).

---

[9] Regulation was interpreted in the broader sense as a legal instrument.

Table 4.2 *Selected aspects of health intelligence for HIA*

	Austria	Belgium	Denmark	England	Finland	Germany	Hungary	Ireland	Italy	Lithuania	Malta	Netherlands	Northern Ireland	Poland	Portugal	Slovakia	Slovenia	Spain	Sweden	Switzerland	Wales
HIA web site				✓	✓		✓				✓	✓	✓						✓		✓
HIA database				✓	✓								✓								✓
HIA review/ overview	✓	✓	✓	✓	✓								✓								✓

An example of a regulation at regional level is the Public Health Service Act of the reference region North Rhine Westphalia in Germany. It provides, in principle, a legal basis for HIA by stating that public health services shall contribute to all planning processes. A similar provision is made in the German state of Saxony-Anhalt.

Selected aspects of health information and intelligence for HIA

Requirements on health information and intelligence can be quite demanding. They may entail availability of information on population health status and health determinants, and if the HIA is conducted at regional and local levels, this information must be available for these levels too.

Apart from data on population health and determinants, health information and intelligence for HIA provide information on the planning and delivery of HIAs including, concepts, methods, tools and evidence. Across all countries, dedicated HIA web sites, HIA databases and HIA reviews or overviews were searched. No distinction was made between levels since it was assumed that health intelligence is a general task which can equally be used at national, regional and local levels (see Table 4.2).

Clearly, in many countries, HIA practitioners have received little support in regard to HIA-related health intelligence. They must rely on their personal experiences and their own networks when planning and conducting HIAs, or they have to use intelligence provided in other countries. However, this may involve problems of transferability.

Box 4.1 *HIA and governance in Wales*

The National Assembly for Wales was established in July 1999. It provides Wales with more control over its own affairs and enables it to set policies to meet its specific needs on a wide range of issues including health. The need to improve health and to reduce health inequalities has been one of its priorities from the outset. Several policy and strategy documents have emphasized the role of all sectors, all levels of government and all parts of society in improving health. Action to support people to take steps to improve their lifestyles is accompanied by wider action across policy areas to tackle social, economic and environmental health determinants. The Welsh Assembly is committed to developing more integrated policies and programmes and, as part of this, to the use of HIA.

HIA is seen as a practical and flexible approach that recognizes the realities and constraints of the planning and decision-making processes involved in the development of policies, programmes and other actions. The initial national guidance document, *Developing health impact assessment in Wales* (National Assembly for Wales, 2000), led to the implementation of a development programme. This included the creation of the Welsh Health Impact Assessment Support Unit. The use of HIA is promoted strongly in national and local policy documents and has a recognized importance within key national and local government bodies. At national level, the Welsh Local Government Association and the National Public Health Service for Wales support the use of HIA and work closely with the support unit. At local level, the 22 local authorities and their corresponding local health boards have a joint statutory duty to develop, implement and evaluate local health, social care and well-being strategies. Guidance issued for the strategies highlighted the role that HIA could play. In support of this, *Improving health and reducing inequalities: a practical guide to health impact assessment* was written by the unit and published by the Welsh Assembly Government in November 2004 (WHIASU, 2004).

The Welsh Health Impact Assessment Support Unit was set up to help organizations and groups outside the Welsh Assembly to understand and use the approach throughout Wales. It has a multifaceted capacity building programme. The Welsh Assembly funds the unit through the Wales Centre for Health, a new independent public body that focuses on addressing inequalities, providing information and advice to the public, developing networks and partnerships, undertaking and commissioning research, and contributing to public health training and education. Funding for the unit covers the costs of two development workers and provides resources for communication and dissemination, including a web site. The unit itself is based in the Cardiff Institute of Society, Health and Ethics in Cardiff University's School of Social Sciences. This maximizes the opportunities for, and links to, academic research alongside the need to develop a practical approach.

Funding and costs of HIA

The following subsection reviews funding arrangements for HIA in the countries included in the research. Information collected on the costs of the HIAs is also presented.

Funding

HIA budgets for sustained funding of support units, centres, institutes and other facilities are scarce, although England, the Republic of Ireland, Northern Ireland, the Netherlands and Wales are exceptions. In some instances, a budget for HIA is reserved within the general budget of national or regional institutes. Funds to conduct HIAs often come from the regular budget of institutes or local administrations.

Budgets for HIAs were reported for eight countries at national level (see Table 4.3). Some reference regions and reference localities have reported budgets. However, they were not included in the table since, for these levels, it was assumed that there were hidden budgets that could not be identified. In most cases, quantification of the budgets was impossible.

There is hardly a common approach between the countries regarding budgets for HIA as the following examples show. The Institute of Public Health in the Republic of Ireland, which provides services for the Republic of Ireland and Northern Ireland, receives funds for the development of HIA from the Irish Department of Health and Children and from the Northern Ireland Department of Health, Social Services and Public Safety. There is a budget for funding the Welsh Health Impact Assessment Support Unit, which is provided by the Welsh Assembly Government. The budget holder is the Wales Centre for Health, a new national body whose main functions are to provide public health information, coordinate the surveillance of health trends and carry out risk assessments of threats to health and well-being, and to train and develop a multidisciplinary public health workforce. In Poland, the Ministry of Health provides funding in the framework of overall political accountability. The budget is held by the chief sanitary inspector. In Slovenia, at national level, the Ministry of Health provides a small budget for HIA for the National Institute of Public Health, defined according to working hours of the staff. However, this budget is not a regular budget but dedicated for special cases.

In England, the Public Health Development Fund provides finances for HIA. For the financial year 1999–2000, £9 million were allocated to support the public health strategy as a whole in areas such as HIA, the development of nine regional Public Health Observatories and the improvement of infection

Table 4.3 *Budgets for HIA at national level*

Austria	Belgium	Denmark	England	Finland	Germany	Hungary	Ireland	Italy	Lithuania	Malta	Netherlands	Northern Ireland	Poland	Portugal	Slovakia	Slovenia	Spain	Sweden	Switzerland	Wales
✓			✓								✓	✓	✓			✓			✓	✓

control (Secretary of State for Health, 1999). Examples of Public Health Observatories' involvement in HIA include the London Health Observatory, which developed a programme of work and had a dedicated HIA facilitator attached to it, and the Yorkshire and Humber Public Health Observatory, which has recently secured funding for a post on health/integrated impact assessment (Hill et al., 2005).

Budgets for HIA were also reported at national and local levels. In the German reference region North Rhine Westphalia, work on HIA is funded as part of the budget of the State Institute of Public Health, which is acting as the state health authority and participating in the financial budget of the State Health Ministry. In Switzerland, a budget comes from the Department of Health and Social Affairs and is managed within the public health office.

At local level in Belgium, the nongovernmental organization (NGO) Leuven Local Agenda 21 was reported as a budget holder for HIA. The budget comes from the City Council, which in turn receives its funds from different sources, such as the Flemish Government, the Government of the Province of Vlaams-Brabant and from the funds of cities and communities. For municipalities in Germany, the local health authority's budget is responsible for funding. In Finland, the city of Jyväskylä held the project budget. Box 4.2 discusses HIA financing in the Netherlands.

Costs of an HIA

It has been argued that the costs of an HIA can be very high and this might constitute a problem, especially in a situation when it is unclear who will bear the burden (Krieger et al., 2003). Furthermore, the costs of an HIA must be proportional to the decision at hand (Atkinson & Cooke, 2005). Different types of HIA require different analytical methods, and provision for participation costs can vary considerably between individual HIAs. A mini or desktop HIA will certainly consume far less resources than a maxi or comprehensive HIA. Therefore, a differentiated picture of the type of HIA and

Box 4.2 *Financing HIA: the Netherlands*

The attention to HIA in the Netherlands can be separated into two periods. The first is from 1996 to 2003. In 1996, the Ministry of Health, Welfare and Sports installed an Intersectoral Policy Office at the National School of Public Health. This office was the governmental agency that was responsible for commissioning experimental HIAs on national policy proposals and developing HIA methodology, including building a network of relevant organizations for HIA. The Ministry of Health allocates a part of its budget to the Intersectoral Policy Office. The annual budget increased from €230 000 in 1996 to €340 000 in 2001.

The second period started in 2003 when the Ministry of Health decided to stop the funding to the Intersectoral Policy Office and to start funding a number of connected research projects together with the funding of projects to support municipalities. As a result, a part of the function of the Intersectoral Policy Office was taken over by the National Institute of Public Health and the Environment, including research and the networking function, e.g. organizing meetings in which health impact screening and related topics are discussed. Until 2006, a budget was available for maintaining intersectoral policy in the work of the National Institute of Public Health and the Environment. In addition, funds are available for two PhD studies on HIA. One focuses on the development of instruments for analysing and influencing administrative processes in the interests of public health and the other focuses on the development of instruments for analysing and quantifying the impact of policy on public health.

the costs incurred would be welcome. Unfortunately, despite the growing interest in evaluation of HIA, very little information on the costs of HIAs is available.

Among the few examples currently available are those presented in the "Merseyside Guidelines". On the basis of three projects, the calculated average cost of an HIA was €18 000,[10] of which €15 000 represented the actual costs of assessor/support staff time[11] (Scott-Samuel, Birley & Ardern, 1998). The costs of the Finningley Airport HIA, which was concluded in 2000, were calculated at €76 000 to €101 000 in actual staff costs and €25 000 for commissioning and disseminating (Abdel Aziz, Radford & McCabe, 2004). The costs of the HIA of Dulwich Healthy Living Centre, which was concluded in 2003, were calculated at €36 000 (Atkinson & Cooke, 2005).

Among the 158 HIAs identified and analysed in the project, information on the costs incurred was only available in 15 cases (see Table 4.4).

---

[10] All figures in this paragraph were converted to euro and rounded off.
[11] The calculation was based on (i) actual costs of the person–hours input of assessors and of administrative/secretarial staff; (ii) notional costs of the person–hours input of academic staff, Steering Group members and key informants; and (iii) notional travel expenses.

Box 4.3 *Capacity building for HIA in the Republic of Ireland and Northern Ireland*

The Institute of Public Health was established in 1999 to promote cooperation for public health in Northern Ireland and the Republic of Ireland. It aims to improve health across the whole island by working to combat health inequalities and influence public policies in favour of health. A substantial work programme on HIA has been developed in response to needs identified by the health departments and health practitioners in both jurisdictions.

The aim is to promote the implementation of HIA across the island and act as a resource to support government departments, health services and other agencies involved with HIA.

The Institute is currently the only organization on the island providing comprehensive training in HIA. The three-day course furnishes participants with the practical skills necessary to conduct HIA and provides networking opportunities for organizations working within different structures in Northern Ireland and the Republic of Ireland. Shorter "awareness raising" and "taster" sessions are also held for those who wish to increase their knowledge of HIA.

A number of resources for HIA in the Republic of Ireland have been developed by the Institute, including a practical guidance manual and reviews of the links between transport and health, and employment and health. A dedicated HIA web site provides information on the concept and practice of HIA across the island as well as links to international developments in HIA and other useful sites. The Institute coordinates an HIA network and members receive a quarterly newsletter.

The Institute collaborates with organizations throughout the island as well as international partners in building capacity for HIA.

Capacity building

Capacity building provides specific input for the HIA system. Key aspects are the production and training of HIA practitioners, and the establishment of support units. There can be a close link between capacity building and health intelligence, since support units may provide health intelligence required for conducting HIA. Box 4.3 provides a detailed example for the republic of Ireland and Northern Ireland.

Table 4.5 presents aggregated data on the organizations and institutions involved in resource generation. The row total exceeds the number of countries included in the research, since in some countries a multitude of organizations and institutions are involved in capacity building. The absence of resource generation and capacity building was only reported from one

Table 4.4 Costs of an HIA[a]

Country	Year	Level	Type	Sector	Topic	Costs (€)
Belgium	2001	Regional	Maxi/comprehensive	Transport	Noise, pollution, stress	€25000
	2004	Regional	Standard/intermediate	Environment	Pollution	€20000
Lithuania	2004	Local	Standard/intermediate	Multisectoral	Noise, pollution, waste, stress, working environment	€4600
Northern Ireland	2002	Regional	Standard/intermediate	Social care	Access to information and services	€29000
Ireland	2004	Local	Maxi/comprehensive	Transport	Traffic	€63000 available[b]
	2004	Local	Standard/intermediate	Housing/urban planning	Local area plan	€10000
Slovenia	1994	Local	Standard/intermediate	Energy	Pollution	€10000
	1994	Local	Mini/desktop	Housing/urban planning	Other pollution, contamination, infestation	€1000
	1998	Local	Mini/desktop	Tourism	Other bathing water pollution	€2000
	1997	Local	Mini/desktop	Industry	Other noise pollution, air and water pollution	€2000
	2004	Local	Mini/desktop	Industry	Pollution	€5500
Wales	2000	Local	Maxi/comprehensive	Employment	Housing, economic	€33000[c]
	1999	Local	Maxi/comprehensive	Transport	Pollution	€81000[d]
	2002	Local	Maxi/comprehensive	Housing/urban planning	Noise, stress, living conditions	€7000
	2001	Local	Maxi/comprehensive	Housing/urban planning	Community change, health, well-being, housing, indoor air quality, environment	€145000[e]

[a] Domestic currencies were converted into euros and sums were rounded.
[b] Part of the HIA was the production of 65 000 two-page summary leaflets for distribution to local households. €10 000 is allocated to evaluation.
[c] A social and health impact assessment involved questionnaires to be completed by all households.
[d] The total cost was spent over a 3-year period. Methods included questionnaires, diaries, lung function tests and measurement of air pollutant levels.
[e] The high costs of the Welsh impact assessment may relate to the methodology. Apart from the use of routine data, detailed health data was collected from 300 households one year prior to the renovation, shortly before the renovation and after the renovation. The modelling of the community used a sophisticated geographical information system.

Table 4.5 *Resource generation and capacity building: organizations and institutions involved*

	Government	Government agency	NGO	Public health association	University	Other	None
National levels	4	5	6	1	12	8	1
Reference regions	13	14	7	7	6	7	2
Reference localities	5	7	6	1	8	4	1

country at national, two countries at regional and one country at local level.[12] The table demonstrates the multitude of organizations and institutions involved. The involvement of governments, government agencies and universities were frequently reported.

Again, the data at subnational level need to be interpreted with great care, since only a single reference region and a single reference locality were included in the research.

Sweden serves as an example for the complementary roles of different institutions in resource generation and capacity building. The Swedish National Institute for Public Health is developing the methodology for conducting HIAs at local, regional and national levels using the Gothenburg consensus framework as a model. Ongoing projects include:

- supporting governmental agencies within different sectors to implement HIA in their work;

- HIA as a methodology for social sustainable regional development;

- developing HIA methodology for municipalities;

- conducting case studies on road projects, 3G and climate change.

General education on HIA is a subject of public health courses given at different universities, for example Karolinska Institute and Malmö University College. The Swedish Association of Local Authorities and Regions has developed an instrument "Focusing on Health", which can be found on the web site of WHO Regional Office for Europe.

The roles may vary in scope. An example is the government's involvement in Malta. The Office of the Director General of Health took responsibility for

---

[12] The calculation was based on (i) actual costs of the person–hours input of assessors and of administrative/secretarial staff; (ii) notional costs of the person–hours input of academic staff, Steering Group members and key informants; and (iii) notional travel expenses.

introducing the concept of HIA during the period of accession by introducing training both in Malta and abroad. However, according to the data presented in Chapter 3, this has not yet led to a large number of HIAs.[13]

Delivering

Four aspects of the delivery function of HIA systems were analysed. First, "lead agencies" for HIA were identified. A lead agency is defined as the focal point that may also exert technical leadership. This could entail conducting, organizing, managing, commissioning or supervising the HIA. Second, who actually conducted the assessment was analysed. Third, the link between the owners of a pending decision and the triggering of the HIA process were explored. Finally, the link between the assessment and the reporting of the results were analysed. The latter two issues already refer to institutionalization of HIA since they imply the integration of the HIA in the decision-making process.

Lead agencies are established in most countries

On the basis of the project data, four major observations regarding the lead agency can be made.

First, with Austria and Portugal as the only exception (data for Portugal are incomplete), each country identified lead agencies. This is in itself unsurprising, since almost all countries in the sample have a policy, a regulation or other means of endorsement in place establishing the case for HIA.

Second, for most countries and their reference regions and reference localities, lead agencies have been identified on all relevant levels. In only five countries no lead agency was identified for more than one of the relevant levels. It was taken into account that due to the differences in political, administrative and institutional settings some countries have only two relevant levels.

Third, in nine countries the function of the lead agency was shared on the same level between different entities. The data were not detailed enough to determine if these lead agencies were conducting their tasks in a complementary, overlapping or conflicting manner.

Fourth, there are a multitude of different bodies and entities serving the function as a lead agency; however, a key role is played by governments and the public sector administration or institutes. Governments as lead agencies

---

[13] However, in some countries one of the levels was not applicable due to the institutional setting.

were specifically identified at national and local levels. This was the case with 11 countries. In six of them, both national and local governments were identified as lead agencies and frequently the public sector administration or institutes were identified as the lead agency. However, they were exclusively located at national and local levels. Public health associations were identified in six countries as lead agencies, universities or their respective units in six cases, and NGOs in three countries. Other lead agencies were identified in four cases, exclusively located at local level.

Conducting the HIA

The analysis of who conducted the assessment of the HIA has produced a multitude of assessors. Variations are considerable. Quite often assessment is conducted by a combination of assessors, or the assessors are supported by other organizations, groups and individuals. A case study for Lithuania is provided in Box 4.4.

Examples from the local level in Finland have shown that variations regarding the choice of assessors may be found at the same level. In one exceptional case, the HIA was performed by students of Turku Polytechnic. In many other cases, the assessment was conducted by the responsible planner from the city administration itself, with the support of the National Research and Development Centre for Welfare and Health (STAKES). In two cases, it was the local Energy and Waste Management Corporation. These assessments were conducted by external consultants.

For England, data on who has conducted HIAs are only available for 9 of the selected 28 HIAs. It was either the entity that triggered the HIA process or independent consultants; 19 local HIAs were reported for Wales. A multitude of groups, organizations and institutions have been involved in triggering and conducting the HIAs in Wales. Historically, local health authorities supported HIAs. More recently, the Welsh Assembly, local authorities and local health boards, with the support of the Welsh Health Impact Assessment Support Unit in some cases, have taken on this role. Many of the HIAs have been collaborative undertakings, with local health alliances playing an important part. For one of the HIAs reported in Belgium, the policy was owned by Leuven City Council. The HIA was triggered by a partnership of 25 institutions, business organizations and citizens' groups and the HIA was conducted jointly by the University of Leuven and the Groep T. Leuven Engineering School.

The Italian assessment on the Brenner motorway was conducted by EURAC (European Academy, Bolzano), a private institute. In Spain, five of the seven

Box 4.4 *Organizations and agencies conducting HIA in Lithuania*

In Lithuania, HIA started in 2004, when two legal acts, foreseen in the Law on Public Health Care (2003) as the supplements for environmental impact assessment (EIA), were approved by the Ministry of Health. In European Union (EU) Member States belonging to the EU before May 2004, HIA is used for the comprehensive assessment of projects, strategies and policies which may have an effect on health at local, regional or national level, and is described as "strategic" HIA. Meanwhile in Lithuania there are a few "strategic" HIAs, and strongly enforced environmental HIA for planned economic activities.

Eighteen institutions (ten public agencies and eight private businesses) were licensed to provide environmental HIA at the State Public Health Service under the Ministry of Health and starting from July 2004 no EIA could be accomplished without a more comprehensive environmental HIA.

From 2001 to 2004, the number of EIAs provided increased from 150 to 422 cases. Most private companies working in the EIA sector tried to obtain their licences for environmental HIA because they saw advantages in this joint action. Furthermore, there is a tendency for public health professionals to shift their positions from governmental public health agencies to private consultancy companies as this is an easier way to coordinate projects and reports with public health institutions.

HIAs identified were part of an EIA and followed the legal requirements. However, a fifth was identified which was initiated by the Public Health Agency of Barcelona. It was conducted by L. Agència de Salut Pública de Barcelona and Mutual Cyclops, Barcelona. In the Netherlands, some of the HIAs were conducted by the Intersectoral Policy Office. Others were conducted by universities or institutes such as SCO Kohnstamm-Institute, the Trimbos-Instituut and The Netherlands Organisation for Applied Scientific Research (TNO), while liaising with the Intersectoral Policy Office.

The link between the pending decision and the HIA

HIAs conducted on an ad hoc basis may sometimes be affected by suspect opportunistic politics. It may be argued that the HIA was only initiated because the expected outcome would support the pending decision. A systematic link between the pending decision and the HIA process may avoid this. The analysis of this link at national level comprised 54 HIAs from 13 countries. Among these HIAs, 18 were from Finland and another 18 from the Netherlands. For the reported cases from Finland, the link was very close. The HIAs, with one exception, were initiated by government departments or government agencies. In the Netherlands, all HIAs were initiated by the Intersectoral Policy Office.

Table 4.6 *Ministries whose policies were the subject of HIAs in the Netherlands and Finland*

Netherlands[a]	Finland
Government	
• Ministry of Finance; Ministry of Health, Welfare and Sports	• Ministry of Agriculture and Forestry
• Ministry of Housing and Spatial Planning	• Ministry of the Environment
• Ministry of Social Affairs and Employment	• Ministry of Trade and Industry
• Ministry of Transport, Public Works and Water Management	• Ministry of Transport and Communication; Prime Minister's Office
• Interdepartmental Commission for Economic and Structural Reinforcement	

[a] *In one case there was not sufficient information to determine who had initiated the HIA.*

They screened the policies of the Ministry of Finance, Ministry of Health, Welfare and Sports, Ministry of Economic Affairs and the Ministry of Housing and Spatial Planning. For all the other countries in the sample, the number of HIAs at national level was too small to report on a pattern.

In the Netherlands, all HIA processes were initiated by the Ministry of Health, Welfare and Sports and the Intersectoral Policy Office. They screen the policies of other ministries for those who might have an impact on health. In practice, the Intersectoral Policy Office plays a major role in this. In Finland, the pattern differs. In general, it is the owner of the policy, programme or project that initiates the HIA process. However, in some cases, working groups were set up that included other ministries or organizations (see Table 4.6).

The link between the pending decision – or the "decision owner" – on the one hand and the initializing of the HIA process on the other was also analysed at regional and local levels. However, the data were less conclusive.

In the selected cases for England there was a close link reported between the owner of the policies, programmes and projects, and the initiation of the HIA. The London Health Commission (LHC) played a key role. It worked in partnership with agencies across the capital to reduce health inequalities and improve the health and well-being of all Londoners. The LHC used HIA to support the development of various Mayor of London strategies: Air Quality, Biodiversity, Children and Young People, Culture, Economic Development, Energy, Noise, Transport, Spatial Development and the London Plan on Waste (LHC, 2005).

A similarly close link at national level is visible for Wales where five HIAs were reported. As a policy owner, the Public Health Strategy Division in the Welsh

Assembly plays an important role in triggering the HIA process and, to a certain degree, is involved in conducting the HIA.

Strategic HIAs may constitute a slightly different case, since they are not linked to a decision. HIAs reported from Germany focused on the health impact of the privatization of drinking water management. In this regard, it was not a reaction to a concrete policy proposal. The lead role in terms of initiating, triggering and conducting the HIA was with the State Institute of Public Health of North Rhine Westphalia in cooperation with the University of Bielefeld (Fehr et al., 2003; Fehr, Mekel & Welteke, 2004).

The link between assessing and reporting

Delivery, as a function of HIA systems, contributes to the achievement of specific HIA objectives. However, if the HIA is not reported adequately to the decision-makers it can neither be taken into consideration nor can it influence the pending decision. In this event, the whole delivery function does not contribute to the objectives of the HIA. This does not exclude other secondary positive effects of an inadequately reported HIA.

As an expansion of the analysis of the stages presented in Chapter 3, the data were analysed in regard to the actual submission of results to the decision-makers.

According to the analysis presented in Table 4.7, reporting back to the policy-makers takes place. However, the data have to be interpreted with great care given the limited availability of data for HIAs at national level and for the reference locality. And, of course, the subnational level was included in the research with only one reference region and one reference locality per country.

The patterns and means of reporting to the decision-makers vary a great deal. According to the data, two major patterns can be distinguished. One is following the formal model of the HIA stages in which the assessment is an activity clearly distinguished from the reporting. Reporting takes place after the assessment has been formally finalized. The other pattern refers to a steady involvement of the decision-makers or their responsible staff. That means that when agreement on the assessment has been achieved no separate or formal reporting is necessary, although written reports may be produced. The means by which the assessment is reported to the decision-makers vary a great deal too. In some cases, submission of the report is the key means of communicating the results. In other cases, individual briefings took place. In several cases, workshops for the decision-maker were organized to inform on the results of the assessment and discuss possible consequences and

Table 4.7 *Reporting to the decision-makers (based on a sample of 158 HIAs)*

	Yes		No		N/A	
	No. of HIAs	%	No. of HIAs	%	No. of HIAs	%
National level	27	50.0	11	20.4	16	29.6
Reference region	14	65.2	7	30.4	2	4.3
Reference locality	31	38.3	26	32.1	24	29.6

options. Some HIAs have used a combination of means for reporting to the decision-makers.

As Table 4.7 suggests, in a fair number of cases within the sample of HIAs analysed, the results of the assessment were not directly reported to the decision-makers. There are a variety of reasons for this. First, some of the HIAs in this category resembled strategic HIAs. Decision-makers were involved in them and they were linked to the broader policy process but not to a specific pending decision. The explicit role of the HIA was to prepare a public debate on future directions in a specific policy field. However, there are other cases in which there was no link with the decision-makers. One reason for this was that the assessment was not finalized on time. Interrelating the HIA stages and the policy cycle was unsuccessful. A second reason for not reporting directly to the decision-makers was an obvious disinterest of the decision-makers in the HIA. A third reason was that some of the HIAs were conducted as a scientific project which was eventually published in a scientific journal but was never intended to be reported to the decision-makers.

Conclusion

This mapping exercise has provided evidence that most countries have been implementing HIA at least on a project basis. Implementation takes a variety of forms and varies considerably from country to country. Although governments and government agencies play an important role in the implementation and delivery of HIA, there is a large variety of other institutions and organizations involved in capacity building and the delivery of HIA including local authorities, public health institutes, health observatories and special HIA units, universities and private companies.

A small number of countries have been able to institutionalize HIA at least partially. England, Finland, the Netherlands and Wales should be mentioned in this context. Important elements of this institutionalization are comparable strong governance support as illustrated by the Welsh case study (Case study

9), the establishment of dedicated support units or explicitly integrating responsibilities for HIA in existing institutions, developing the health intelligence for HIA and regular funding for HIA activities. The analysis of the link between the pending proposal, the HIA and the decision-making process has provided examples that HIA can be conducted systematically in collaboration with different sectors and departments. However, most countries in the mapping exercise are lacking many of these conditions. Government support is half-hearted, the HIA-related health intelligence is insufficient and funding is provided either on a project basis or from existing resources.

The progress made both in terms of implementation and institutionalization does not necessarily continue. Developments and policy support may vary in the future. This was demonstrated at national level by the case study on the Netherlands. Support for implementation or institutionalization of HIA may dwindle due to changes in governments (Broeder, Penris & Varela Put, 2003). Doubts have also been raised in Germany by the governmental Advisory Council of the Assessments of Developments in Health Care regarding the current knowledge gap and methodological uncertainties and the implementation of HIA (Sachverständigenrat für die Begutachtung der Entwicklung im Gesundheitswesen, 2005). On the other hand it was recently reported that the public health administration of the Swiss Canton Ticino had announced its intention to assess all future political decisions by carrying out an HIA (Danner et al., 2006).

Drawing conclusions regarding the role of HIA as a decision-support tool is difficult due to the limited activities at national level and the small number of HIAs identified at regional level. The evidence suggests that, currently, the strongest developments in HIA are to be observed at local level. Still, the analysis of the link between the pending decision, the HIA and the decision-making process has provided insights that this is possible in principle. In Chapter 2, a summary of the evidence found in the case studies in Parts III, IV and V demonstrates the link between HIA and the decision-making process.

Secondary contributors to this chapter

Elisabet Aldenberg, Swedish National Institute of Public Health, Sweden; Franz Baro, WHO Collaborating Centre on Health and Psychosocial Factors, Belgium; Francisco Barroso Martin, Técnicas de Salud S.A., Spain; Ceri Breeze, Welsh Assembly Government, Wales, United Kingdom; Konrade von Bremen, Institute of Health Economics and Management, Switzerland; Edit Eke, Semmelweis University, Hungary; Rainer Fehr, LÖGD (Landesinstitut für den Öffentlichen Gesundheitsdienst) NRW, Germany; Mojca Gabrijelčič Blenkuš, Institute of Public Health of the Republic of Slovenia; Gabriel Gulis,

University of Southern Denmark, Denmark; Tapani Kauppinen, National Research and Development Centre for Welfare and Health (STAKES), Finland; Jarmila Korcova, Trnava University, Slovakia; Odile Mekel, LÖGD, Germany; Owen Metcalfe, The Institute of Public Health, Ireland; Kirsi Nelimarkka, STAKES, Finland; José Pereira-Miguel, University of Lisbon, Portugal; Kerttu Perttilä, STAKES, Finland; Walter Riccardi, Institute of Hygiene, Catholic University of the Sacred Heart, Rome, Italy; Martin Sprenger, Medical University of Graz, Austria; Ingrid Stegeman, EuroHealthNet, Belgium; Lorraine Taylor, former Health Development Agency, United Kingdom; Rudolf Welteke, LÖGD, Germany; Cezary Wlodarczyk, CM Jagiellonian University, Poland.

REFERENCES

Abdel Aziz MI, Radford J, McCabe J (2004). The Finningley Airport HIA: a case study. In: Kemm J, Parry J, Palmer S, eds. *Health impact assessment.* Oxford, Oxford University Press: 285–298.

Danner G, et al., eds (2006). Schweiz: Politik überprüft sich selbst [Switzerland: Government reviews policies]. *EUREPORT social*, 14(3):17.

Atkinson P, Cooke A (2005). Developing a framework to assess costs and benefits of health impact assessment. *Environmental Impact Assessment Review*, 25(7–8):791–798.

Banken R (2001). *Strategies for institutionalizing HIA.* Brussels, WHO Regional Office for Europe.

Banken R (2003). Health impact assessment – how to start the process and make it last. *Bulletin of the World Health Organization*, 81(6):389.

Broeder LD, Penris M, Varela Put G (2003). Soft data, hard effects. Strategies for effective policy on health impact assessment – an assessment analysis and procedures in the European experience. *Bulletin of the World Health Organization*, 81(6):404–407.

Department of Health (2004). *Choosing health: making healthy choices easier. Executive summary.* London, Department of Health.

Fehr R et al. (2003). Towards health impact assessment of drinking-water privatization – the example of waterborne carcinogens in North Rhine-Westphalia (Germany). *Bulletin of the World Health Organization*, 81(6):408–414.

Fehr R, Mekel O, Welteke R (2004). HIA: the German perspective. In: Kemm J, Parry J, Palmer S, eds. *Health impact assessment.* Oxford, Oxford University Press:253–264.

Hill A, et al. (2005). Building public health skills and capacity in the English regions. *Public Health*, 119(4):235–238.

Kemm J (2005a). HIA – growth and prospects. *Environmental Impact Assessment Review*, 25(7–8):691–692.

Kemm J (2005b). The future challenges for HIA. *Environmental Impact Assessment Review*, 25(7–8):799–807.

Krieger N, et al. (2003). Assessing health impact assessment: multidisciplinary and international perspectives. *Journal of Epidemiology and Community Health*, 57:659–662.

LHC (2005). *What is the London Health Commission?* London, London Health Commission (http://www.londonshealth.gov.uk/pdf/whatisthelhc.pdf, accessed 24 April 2006).

National Assembly for Wales (2000). *Developing health impact assessment in Wales: better health better Wales.* Cardiff, National Assembly for Wales.

Sachverständigenrat für die Begutachtung der Entwicklung im Gesundheitswesen (2005). Koordination und Qualität im Gesundheitswesen, Bd I: *Kooperative Koordination und Wettbewerb, Sozioökonomischer Status und Gesundheit, Strategien der Primärprävention [Cooperative coordination and competition, socio-economic status and health, strategies for prevention].* Stuttgart, Nomos.

Saltman RB, Ferrousier-Davis O (2000). The concept of stewardship in health policy. *Bulletin of the World Health Organization*, 78(6):732–739.

Scott-Samuel A, Birley M, Ardern K (1998). *Merseyside guidelines for health impact assessment.* Liverpool, Merseyside Health Impact Assessment Steering Group/Liverpool Public Health Observatory.

Secretary of State for Health (1999). *Saving lives: our healthier nation* (Vol. Cm 4386). London, The Stationery Office.

Ståhl T, et al. (2006). Health in all policies: prospects and potentials. Helsinki, Ministry of Social Affairs and Health (Finland).

Travis P, et al. (2003). Towards better stewardship: concepts and critical issues. In: Murray CJL, Evans DB, eds. *Health systems performance assessment: methods, debate and empiricism.* Geneva, World Health Organization:289–300.

WHIASU (2004). *Improving health and reducing inequalities: a practical guide to health impact assessment.* Cardiff, Welsh Health Impact Assessment Support Unit, Welsh Assembly Government.

WHO (2000). *Health systems: improving performance.* Geneva, World Health Organization.

Part III
The Effectiveness of Health Impact Assessment: Case Studies

Case study 1

A large-scale urban development HIA: focusing on vulnerable groups in London, England

Katie Collins and Lorraine Taylor[1]

Introduction

This case study details the process and effectiveness of the King's Cross health impact assessment (HIA), which had the task of considering six major developments taking place over 20 years in the King's Cross area of London.

In order to create this case study, four interviews were conducted with the following participants in the HIA: a decision-maker, an HIA administrator, an HIA practitioner and a stakeholder. A group discussion was conducted with six community members and community workers in HIA.

The King's Cross HIA has two specific characteristics. The first is its size, scope and duration. This HIA deals with six major construction projects and could be extended until 2020 when the construction projects are planned to end. It also has local, regional, national and international dimensions. The second is that it concerns particularly vulnerable communities and socially excluded groups who live in and around King's Cross. These may be impacted adversely not only by the construction works but also by the effects of gentrification of the area.

---

[1] With particular thanks to all the participants involved in this case study.

The scope of the HIA

Four transport infrastructure developments and two mixed-use developments were examined (King's Cross Central and Regent's Quarter). The majority of the work was conducted by the HIA between September 2002 and November 2005.

The HIA provided direct evidence for the two following decisions: the Channel Tunnel Rail Link (CTRL) planning enquiry into 24-hour working in January 2004 and the developers' application for planning permission for the King's Cross Central Development. This consisted of responses to several documents and two stages of planning applications for Camden Primary Care Trust (PCT) and Islington PCT between 2002 and 2005. The final planning decision was made in March 2006.

There were separate decision-making alternatives for each construction project. The transport construction projects were covered by the Provider Sponsored Act of Parliament (TSO, 1996) and decisions could be made about the construction process only, not the nature of the construction plans. In addition, CTRL and Regent's Quarter had already been under development when the HIA started and therefore it was able to influence decisions only on works taking place. The King's Cross Central development had not received planning consent when the HIA began. The PCTs' input was concerned with modifying the plans to the benefit of the health of the community, rather than preventing the development.

The HIA took into account the national and international implications of the redevelopments, considering their effects on the local population of 17 000 to 23 000 people comprising many vulnerable groups. The completed development will have at least 3000 new residents and 35 000 workers on site, as well as an anticipated 5 million visitors (including tourists) per year. The HIA had to take into account not only the health effects on the existing community but also the potential health needs of this new community and the strain that this growth in population could impose on local primary care and hospital services. In addition, the disruption caused by construction works and potential gentrification of the area were predicted to have the potential to displace sex workers and drug users to other areas of Camden, which may correspondingly affect the health of people living in these areas.

The study also had to consider the London-wide impacts of what is understood to be the largest construction site in Europe and the potential for migration from other areas of the country to King's Cross once the construction is completed. King's Cross is a major transport hub: 68 million passenger journeys a year are predicted to pass through it by 2018. The CTRL will also bring international travellers and residents to the area, therefore the study could be said to have an international dimension.

Geographical and social settings

The area in which the HIA took place is in central London, identified in Camden PCT's HIA response to the Argent St George planning application as sitting "on the boundary of the two most deprived boroughs in London". It also states that King's Cross and Somers Town are among the most deprived 20% of wards in England. Unemployment is 7–13%, but much higher for black and ethnic minority groups in the community. About half of the households in the King's Cross area have an income of less than £200 per week. There is an acute need for housing in the area: Camden is ranked as the seventh most crowded borough in England. Access to primary health care is poor, especially for black and minority ethnic (BME) communities, and 23% of residents have difficulties coping with daily life (General Health Questionnaire (GHQ) score of 4+) to the extent that they may be suffering from psychiatric morbidity.

The HIA was commissioned on behalf of Camden and Islington PCTs and organized by them at the local level. They provided the main funding, with additional funding from King's Cross Partnership for Urban Regeneration. The driving force behind the HIA was the Director of Public Health at Camden PCT.

The development straddles both Camden and Islington Borough Councils. Their respective PCTs had to work together to submit responses to various decisions about proposed and current construction projects at King's Cross. This was made easier by the close links engendered between Islington and Camden when they were part of one PCT.

The Director of Public Health at Camden PCT had a high profile and was generally respected, making it easier to attract funding and participation in the HIA. The HIA gained some kudos when this person moved on to public health work at a national level during the course of the HIA.

Model

The HIA followed the model defined in the Gothenburg consensus (European Centre for Health Policy, 1999) and in *Health Impact Assessment* (Kemm, Parry & Palmer, 2004a). The rapid appraisal techniques used follow the outline developed for the Faculty of Public Health (Ison, 2002) and the techniques outlined in the chapter on rapid appraisal techniques in *Health Impact Assessment* (Kemm, Parry & Palmer, 2004b).

The techniques outlined in *Planning for Real* (e.g. Gibson, 1998) helped to inform the content of the rapid appraisal workshops. However, this HIA was also reactive and innovative in its approach, developing new models of community consultation as a result of inadequate contact with hard-to-reach groups in the community during the initial rapid appraisal phase.

The HIA was divided into three different phases. The preparatory phase took place between April and September 2002 and involved a literature review, needs assessment, baseline data, scoping and establishment of the steering group.

Phase 1 took place between October 2002 and summer 2003. This used rapid appraisal techniques in two large series of consultation events with stakeholders including participatory stakeholder workshops, open events for the community and business forums. Results were collated and analysed to help inform the planning process in the following key areas: community; BME groups; construction impacts; emergency planning; economic issues; social and cultural issues; amenities, facilities and services; housing and environment; transport.

Phase 2 took place between February and August 2004. This involved a further consultation with stakeholders, particularly hard-to-reach groups, using in-depth techniques and monitoring trends relating to health and well-being.

Actors

At the beginning of the project Camden PCT put together an HIA team with responsibility for coordinating the HIA and setting the parameters of enquiry and approach. A steering group met quarterly to discuss the direction of the HIA and plan future action. This comprised a diverse group of decision-makers, members of Camden and Islington PCTs, developers' representatives and other local stakeholders. It enabled the development of personal networks and encouraged communication. There was generally good attendance at the sessions. The HIA team and the steering group could also call on a pool of individuals with specific expertise on an ad hoc basis.

HIA reports and information were disseminated to many stakeholder groups in the boroughs of Camden and Islington, including residents, local businesses, MPs, the police and local charities via email, post, presentations and invitations to participate in workshops.

Community workers in community engagement

At the end of the first round of rapid-appraisal workshops it was felt that several communities suffering from health inequalities had been underrepresented. It was decided that community workers should be employed to consult such hard-to-reach groups. This methodology was characterized as innovative and ground-breaking by those working in the HIA and the community workers themselves.

Voluntary Action Camden employed 10 members of the local community, recruited through posters, advertisements in local publications and word of mouth in the King's Cross area. Pre-employment interviews revealed that many of the workers had previous experience of working within the 10 hard-to-reach groups that they set out to interview: the Bangladeshi community; Turkish-speaking community; young people; women sex workers and drug users/ex-drug users; Somali community; families with children; refugees and asylum seekers; homeless people; older people; wheelchair users and people with visual impairments.

The community workers were trained in HIA interview techniques and attended a workshop on report writing. They undertook consultations in the form of workshops, in-depth interviews and discussions with community members; produced information materials to enable people to make informed comments and prepared individual reports for their sectors.

This Community Workers in HIA (CWHIA) project was informed and overseen by an additional steering group made up of representatives from local voluntary organizations and action groups, as well as some members of Camden and Islington PCTs. HIA members reported the progress of this steering group and the community workers to the guidance group. The project was funded from neighbourhood renewal funding disbursed by Camden Central Community Umbrella (CCCU), matched in equal amounts by Camden and Islington PCTs.

Aims of the HIA

The scoping document clearly stated that the aim of the HIA is to identify the redevelopment's potential impacts on health and well-being and highlight ways in which to reduce negative and enhance positive impacts; maximize opportunities for health gain; present recommendations based on the findings of the HIA to various organizations and decision-makers involved in, or affected by, the redevelopment; involve the community in the process and consider the most appropriate means of monitoring the impacts of construction on people's health and well-being.

Dimensions of effectiveness

It is difficult to assess the effectiveness of the King's Cross HIA for several reasons. The criteria that have been set for the evaluation are not identical to the aims set by the HIA itself and, while it may have been effective in its own terms, it may not be as effective against the criteria set by this project. The HIA was one of many inputs into the decision-making process. Many people mentioned a lack of information about concrete examples of the HIA's influence on decision-making. In addition, the effects of some of the decisions which it informed have not been realized, for example, King's Cross Central has not been built yet.

Health effectiveness

Most people agreed that the HIA was most directly effective in terms of health. The decision not to allow 24-hour working at King's Cross Central and the ensuing health benefits to the community were attributed directly to the PCTs' evidence at the planning enquiry. In addition, the problems identified with emergency planning and the subsequent changes in the planning proposals were attributed directly to the HIA. The primary care provision that is anticipated to be included in the Section 106 (Town and Country Planning Act, 1990) agreement is also felt to affect directly the health of the community and of passengers passing through King's Cross.

In addition to this direct health effectiveness, there was a sense that the HIA had created an awareness of the wider determinants of health that may influence decision-makers. It was also noted that the information provided by the HIA could enable the PCTs to negotiate a number of measures to improve the health of their communities, if they so wish.

Equity effectiveness

The HIA was seen to be more generally effective in relation to equity. The decision not to allow 24-hour working was seen as directly effective as it affected the most economically disadvantaged members of the local community who live in an estate very close to the construction works. However, there were very few other examples of the effectiveness of direct equity.

Several participants felt that the HIA consultation process gave people a new way to express their wants and needs, and that the idiom of health carried more weight with developers and decision-makers than simply asking for things. Groups such as drug users, homeless people and sex workers could be included on an equal footing with other community members, because no one could deny their right to good health.

On the whole, the HIA was thought to have contributed to an environment where decision-makers were sensitized to the equity needs of disadvantaged and hard-to-reach groups. The HIA's efforts to contact these groups also encouraged other actors and institutions involved in the development to take a similar approach. However, some participants noted that consultation does not necessarily result in decisions that increase equity. There was some suspicion that certain decisions that appear to increase equity will lose out to the competing demands of those with more social capital.

Community effectiveness

One participant mentioned that two community members had approached the Director of Public Health to voice concerns about the effects of the construction works on the health of the community and that this intervention was a driving force behind the commissioning of the HIA. The fact that the HIA was in some part prompted by the actions of community members points to direct community effectiveness.

The CWHIA project was seen as an opportunity to train community members in facilitation techniques and to set up a community enterprise at the end of the process, producing a tangible community benefit. This benefit was emphasized by most of the participants, who also underlined the innovative and ground-breaking nature of the project. However, the long-term benefit was not as extensive as expected because there was only enough funding for two community workers to set up a social enterprise at the end of the project.

The HIA community consultation process was a vehicle for informing the local community about the extent and duration of the construction projects and managed to include a number of hard-to-reach groups that had not been consulted. Many had not been aware that construction works would last until 2020.

Community members took knowledge gained from the HIA into other consultations and used it to argue their points. One particular example cited was community members' contribution to the King's Cross Developers Forum set up by the council to mediate between the developers and the community. However, community effectiveness has been undermined by the lack of feedback to participants in the consultation and the community workers. The lack of resolution or evidence of effectiveness could make the community reluctant to participate in a similar exercise.

Drivers of effectiveness

The effectiveness of the HIA was influenced positively by the involvement of the PCTs and strong leadership at the start. Also, the HIA's commitment to comprehensive community consultation made it of interest to local politicians and community-action groups. Another key driver of effectiveness was the rolling nature of the HIA which allowed it to address several planning decisions over a number of years.

Role of the PCTs

The HIA was commissioned by the local PCTs which caused some funding issues for such a large-scale and long-running HIA. However, this was also a strength as the PCTs provided an existing body of knowledge about the issues in the area and were able to focus on relevant health impacts in an efficient and effective way.

The strong historical links between Camden and Islington PCTs have been noted already. The King's Cross developments span both boroughs and therefore it was essential that the administrations in both boroughs work together and support the HIA. This process was facilitated by each PCT funding an officer to liaise between the PCTs, local authority and community stakeholders.

The HIA was most effective when it had strong backing and leadership from both external consultants and influential staff within the PCTs. The steering group comprised members of various stakeholder groups, including key decision-makers, local councillors and those initially sceptical about the role of the HIA. This meant that it was able to promote an understanding of the socioeconomic determinants of health among several key actors. However, this steering group was brought together only by the influence of key members of staff within the PCTs.

Community consultation

The use of innovative methodologies of community consultation improved the community effectiveness of the HIA, gaining the views of hard-to-reach audiences and disseminating information throughout the community. Members of the PCTs' HIA team employed and trained community members to take an active role in consulting members of hard-to-reach groups in their own community. This approach to community consultation increased the effectiveness of the HIA in gathering evidence from those who are most affected by health inequalities and meant that their voices were represented in recommendations that informed planning decisions.

Long-term HIA

The rolling nature of the HIA ensured that the PCTs had a body of evidence to consult for each new planning decision and did not have to start from a blank slate each time.

The HIA team not only responded to individual planning applications, but also was able to try to influence the decision-making process on a higher level by contributing to context analysis documents for Islington PCT and planning and development documents for Camden PCT. This was a key driver in Camden PCT's success in arguing against 24-hour working, creating good publicity for the HIA and thereby driving other areas of success.

Barriers to effectiveness

The key barriers to effectiveness related to the problems of conducting such a wide-ranging and long-running HIA. In addition, while the HIA made great efforts to include as many groups as possible in the process, this also led to problems of communication about the role of the HIA and in managing the expectations of different groups. The ground-breaking and experimental nature of the CWHIA project also led to some problems in communicating the outcomes of this project effectively and to a wide audience.

Problems of conducting a long-running HIA

Over the course of the HIA a number of staff changes affected its status in local government and PCT structures. One participant noted that this change of PCT staff coincided with an apparent change of priorities, with more emphasis on primary care and a more medical definition of the HIA's remit.

Staff changes at the PCTs made it difficult for the HIA to maintain momentum and high levels of influence with decision-makers. In addition, it contributed to the difficulty in obtaining continued funding, limiting the resources available for researching the health impacts of the construction works and finished projects. This undermined the scientific validity of the HIA's evidence and recommendations, having a directly negative effect on the effectiveness of the HIA's influence on decision-making.

The lack of HIA resolution or any publicity about decisions it had influenced were significant barriers to community effectiveness in particular. Indeed, these created disaffection with the consultation process within the community and may reduce their willingness to participate in similar consultations.

Reconciling the needs of different stakeholders

Another key barrier to the effectiveness of the HIA was the difficulty of reconciling the needs and priorities of different stakeholders. One participant noted that several of the institutions involved in the HIA had difficulty negotiating the socioeconomic determinants of health and incorporating the HIA recommendations into their decision-making structures.

The need for an affordable supermarket providing high-quality food was mentioned as one recommendation that could not be incorporated in the planning decision as it does not include that kind of detail. This was used as an example of the need for a process of translation between the concepts of the HIA and those of other institutions.

It was mentioned that the developers in particular found it difficult to adapt to a socioeconomic model of health because they were more focused on measurable effects such as air quality. While it was felt that this had improved to some extent, fundamental structural changes in institutions would need to take place for the socioeconomic determinants of health to be incorporated fully into decision-making.

Role and nature of the HIA

Some stakeholders, particularly community members, were unclear about the role and limitations of the HIA. Two participants noted that the community was not always clear what the HIA was, or what its aims were. Community consultation was kept separate from other work leading some community members to believe that this was the entire HIA. This meant that people may have had unrealistic expectations and may point to the need to manage expectations in similar exercises.

One participant argued that although the community consultation was a necessary part of the process, it did not provide many insights that were not already being considered. For this person the community consultation was intended to validate the requests in the HIA report, and therefore was successful in this aim. Community workers also suggested that they may have been consulted as a box-ticking exercise rather than because their information was crucial to the HIA.

Experimental nature of community involvement process

Given the experimental nature of this methodology, some aspects of the management of the CWHIA project had a negative effect on the effectiveness of this element of the HIA.

One participant felt that the CWHIA's training period was rather short and intense and not conducted in optimal conditions for community members to learn new skills. They felt that their strengths lay in gathering information rather than organizing it for a professional audience and that this requirement put a lot of stress on them. One required output of the project was for each worker to produce a report for the community they consulted. Community members felt that they were not given adequate training in writing reports of sufficient standard. They asserted that the reports were not published by the PCTs owing to the style in which they were written, which the community workers felt made their contribution less effective. Indeed, one participant felt that they had not been given the emphasis that they merited in the final HIA response to the Argent St George planning application which made little direct reference to the community point of view. It was suggested that publication of the reports had been blocked because they did not fit with the PCT's intended message about the vulnerable communities that were consulted.

Conclusion

This HIA was judged to be somewhat effective in all of the dimensions considered in this study, particularly in terms of health effectiveness with regard to the decision not to allow 24-hour working on the CTRL site. However, it is difficult to assess accurately the effectiveness of the HIA because of its long-running nature, the number of decisions to which it contributed and the fact that several of the developments have not been finished yet.

Several specific characteristics affected the effectiveness and influenced the methods and process of the King's Cross HIA – providing information for a number of different planning and health-care decisions in the area by means of a complex and long-running study. This specific characteristic provided it with opportunities to conduct ongoing research that provided input to a number of different issues. However, it also created challenges in maintaining leadership, funding and momentum. Strategies such as the quarterly HIA steering group helped to drive the HIA but staff changes at the PCTs and difficulties in obtaining funding were barriers to effectiveness.

The HIA was organized on a local level by Camden and Islington PCTs, giving it a strong base of local support and allowing it to take advantage of local health knowledge within the two PCTs. The HIA was championed in Camden PCT by a high-profile and respected individual and this helped to attract funding and the participation of key stakeholders. However, local organization also had disadvantages: it was difficult to maintain funding over a long period, particularly with changes in the PCTs' key staff; and it was challenging to conduct a study of this magnitude.

The HIA made unprecedented attempts to involve the local community, both by informing them of its work and the potential health impacts of the construction project at King's Cross and by training community members in facilitation techniques so that they could engage with hard-to-reach groups. However, community members were uncertain of the usefulness and effectiveness of their input in influencing planning decisions due to the lack of resolution or feedback on the process.

The CWHIA project was intended to empower the community and ensure that the voices of all community members were heard by decision-makers and developers. This project contributed greatly to the community effectiveness of the HIA. However, it also posed some problems for the HIA team in terms of mediating between the realities of the lives and opinions of hard-to-reach community members and the expectations of the PCTs. The difficulty of translation meant that the individual reports of the community workers were not published and therefore these hard-to-reach communities were not represented as strongly as they could have been.

Many lessons can be taken from the evaluation of this HIA to inform future practice for long-term HIAs and models of effective community engagement. The need for continuity of personnel and long-term funding are highlighted by the challenges faced in maintaining momentum, focus and funding. In addition, the innovative methods of community engagement could have been even more effective if accompanied by an ongoing feedback mechanism to explain to community members the effects of community consultation and the wider HIA on influencing development decisions in the area. The CWHIA project would also have been more effective in representing the views of hard-to-reach communities if community workers had been given more help in translating the needs of vulnerable people into language acceptable for a wider audience.

REFERENCES

European Centre for Health Policy (1999). *Health impact assessment: main concepts and suggested approach. Gothenburg consensus paper.* Copenhagen, WHO Regional Office for Europe (http://www. euro.who.int/document/PAE/Gothenburgpaper.pdf [2]).

Gibson T (1998). *The do-ers guide to planning for real exercises.* Telford, Neighbourhood Initiatives Foundation (www.communityplanning.net/methods/method100.htm, accessed 12 June 2006).

Ison E (2002). *Rapid appraisal techniques for health impact assessment.* NICE Faculty of Public Health (PHEL) (http://www.phel.gov.uk/hiadocs/rapidappraisal%20tool_full_document.pdf, accessed 12 June 2006).

---

[2] This reference was provided by one of the interview informants and therefore accessed by the authors of this document.

Kemm J, Parry J, Palmer S, eds (2004a). *Health impact assessment.* Oxford, Oxford University Press.

Kemm J, Parry J, Palmer S (2004b). Rapid appraisal techniques. In: Kemm J, Parry J, Palmer S, eds. *Health impact assessment.* Oxford, Oxford University Press:11–115.

TSO (1990). *Town and Country Planning Act.* London, The Stationery Office. (http://www.opsi.gov.uk/ACTS/acts1996/1996061.htm, accessed 25 March 2007).

TSO (1996). *Channel Tunnel Rail Link Act.* London, The Stationery Office. (http://www.opsi.gov.uk/ACTS/acts1996/1996061.htm, accessed 25 March 2007).

Case study 2

Ecosystem revitalization: community empowerment through HIA in Tuscany, Italy

Roberta Siliquini, Nicola Nante [3] and Walter Ricciardi

Introduction

Political decisions often produce health impacts but sometimes they are difficult to predict. We describe one experience of a health impact assessment (HIA) dealing with the creation of a damp zone that could affect both the ecological system and citizens' health in a rural part of central Italy. This case was chosen because some of the procedures echo those defined as HIA good practice in the international literature. Also, the analysis of potential impact has been completed, allowing some consideration of efficacy and the discussion of limitations and critical points.

When an agricultural firm asked the City Council for permission to create a new damp zone, a year-long HIA was performed in order to inform the decision. The agricultural firm was granted permission with the condition that some post-monitoring procedures were in place.

The assessment activity will be discussed with consideration of context, input and process; particular emphasis will be given to expected and observed effectiveness. The following chapter is based on four interviews with the principal stakeholders and on the reports drafted by the commission (discussed below).

---

[3] Professor Nicola Nante has been involved in the HIA activity as a public health expert.

Profiling HIA activity

HIA culture has solid roots in Italy, thanks to strong care for the environment and the presence of a public health school active since the end of the nineteenth century, but it has not reached the level of development suitable for a tool to help and support policy-makers' decisions.

Despite the fact that many laws (national, regional and local) refer to the attention that policies must pay to health impacts, no law provides HIA as a compulsory or strictly recommended tool.

Similarly, scarce financial resources are allocated ad hoc for this purpose; government agencies rarely develop HIA activities with a stated mission, especially at regional level. Most HIA activities are driven by public or private agencies that provide technical support to institutions in order to help them evaluate their policies. From time to time associations and universities are requested to carry out HIA evaluations, often with different objectives. The majority deal with activity planning and/or research implementation.

We cannot state that there is a real resistance to implementing HIA: the only resistance probably is due to the costs of implementation and the lack of standardized knowledge of the specific topic at overall decision-making and political levels.

At the beginning of 2003, an agricultural firm in Montalcino municipal district asked the City Council for permission to create a wet zone on their land. Montalcino is a rural area, close to Siena in south Tuscany, with low population density. This area is famous for its agricultural production: olive oil and grapes for the vintage Brunello di Montalcino wine.

Land reclamations and agricultural exploitation have reduced significantly Tuscany's previous environment, rich in marshes and ponds. Subsequent neglect and carelessness have seriously compromised the remaining lacustrine areas which are now, for the most part, unproductive and inhospitable even for animals.

The project to restore the wetland deals with requalification programme stated by the agricultural firm's delegate interviewee:

> … Conservation and development of controlled natural areas are able to play an important role for landscape maintenance, and to contrast with the too intensive agricultural use … with all the foreseen benefits of nature, science, education and tourism.

The intended wet zone was a marsh created specifically to build an ecosystem with elevated cultural value by restoring and enlarging it to 20 hectares for public access, and to help attract the fauna that had disappeared.

Permission to restore the wet zone could introduce other benefits:

- creation of a game reserve for hunting stock ducks (a common activity in Tuscany);

- partial deviation of a river course and consequent reallocation of water resources.

The decision about permission to create the wet zone concerned at least two sectors: environment and health. It had to consider any modification to the local ecosystem and the repercussions for the environment such as the entomological problem of the presence of mosquitoes. In order to consider the positives and negatives with regard to environment, health and quality of life, the Mayor nominated a commission to carry out an HIA activity. This was representative of all stakeholders and comprised delegates representing:

- the Mayor

- an agricultural firm

- citizens

- farmers

- science and public health, including an epidemiologist, entomologist and public health professional.

The objectives were to:

- evaluate possible problems deriving from the creation of a wet zone;

- find solutions for minimizing collateral effects on the health of the local population;

- identify direct and indirect costs of managing the wet zone and maintaining the population's good health and quality of life.

The conditions allowed the implementation of a prospective HIA that has been carried out without following an already defined and standardized model. The commission used the following definition of an HIA: "A methodology that allows identification and evaluation of possible changes on a defined population's health, both positive and negative, single or collective, of a procedure/programme/action". Changes taken into consideration can be direct or indirect, occurring within a short- or long-term latency.

At the beginning of 2005 the commission produced the final report. The public health delegate on the commission, a public health professor, stated:

> A correct HIA procedure should take into account the latency
> between the implementation of an intervention and its effects on

health (etiological period). Moreover it requires the availability of the data at the beginning of the intervention and the continuing survey of the health of the population at risk for the whole latency period. As only a preventive evaluation has been planned, our evaluations can have a margin of uncertainty and incompleteness. Anyway the request of the Mayor shows the remarkable sensitivity, far-sightedness and modernity of his approach to citizens' health.

Dimensions of effectiveness

In commissioning the HIA activity, Montalcino Municipality City Council sought to obtain a cost evaluation in terms of risks and long-term benefits of the wet zone project. More specifically, they wanted to gather information about the likely environment and health effects of the wet zone in order to support the Mayor's decision with scientific and objective data. The mayoral delegate on the commission stated: "Each decision, moreover if dealing with a political responsibility, should be characterized by a cost–benefit evaluation."

In order to assess the potential risks for human health, including hypothetical issues and environmental aspects with secondary effects on health and quality of life, the HIA focused on:

- potential risk of infection for humans and domestic animals
- inconveniences due to potential exhalations
- inconveniences due to *Culicidae* (mosquito) infestations
- chemical acute risk (workers' exposure)
- chemical chronic risk (surface water, groundwater, agriculture).

Effectiveness of the HIA activity has been evaluated by analysing the three key dimensions contextualized by the literature: health, equity and community.

Health effectiveness

For health, the HIA addressed all the essential hypothetical aspects in order to avoid unwanted environmental and health-related side-effects. Such side-effects included the association between wet zones and infectious diseases, prevalence of respiratory diseases and prevalence of animal diseases. All the preventive measures of potential threats have been described contextually.

Mosquito control appears to be the most relevant aspect. This should be integrated within the project in the creation and management of the wet zone. Although it is possible to assert that the water depth in the proposed intervention does not produce environmental conditions suitable for mosquito development, health risks are difficult to quantify since they depend in part on the building and management of the project.

The comparative evaluation between the risks and preventive measures has not highlighted particular problems related to creating the wet zone, or whether some important parameters would be monitored. Following the HIA results, a list of parameters was included as an integral part of the resolution to allow the creation of the wet zone. However, the wet zone is very new, and therefore so health impact evaluations of effectiveness have not been implemented yet.

Equity effectiveness

The HIA highlighted how different communities (e.g. agricultural versus suburban communities) were exposed to potential risks in Montalcino Municipality and the area affected by the project. In some areas, the expansion of the damp zone does not necessarily present significant problems for local residents, but in other areas less accustomed to mosquitoes the creation of an artificial damp zone could lead to social conflict.

Guaranteed actions specific to different intensities of risk exposure have been adopted further to the HIA evaluations. Mayoral consent to the creation of the wet zone is conditional upon a *fidejussion* from the agricultural firm. This is a guarantee for any health damages that may affect the most exposed population (including long-term effects) or the need to restore the proposed wet zone to its original environmental condition.

Community effectiveness

We can affirm that HIA activity has helped to develop empowerment of the population. The project area is relatively small, with the population mostly involved in agricultural activities in the same region. With relative geographical isolation and strict links of social relations, they must be considered communities with a high information exchange level. The small size of the municipal population increases the likelihood of high civic involvement in council decisions, as the City Council is elected by this same population.

HIA implementation has enabled the population to be aware of scientific and not subjective evaluations of the socioeconomic repercussions of the wet zone project. It has also stimulated a higher concern and attention for future public decisions and a better modulation of interventions. For instance, the community is now more aware of the risks of mosquitoes. As a result they have focused more on these issues in urban areas and stimulated the City Council to adopt the proper interventions.

The implementation of HIA activity led to unexpected administrative and economic results. As a programmed activity with fixed costs it eliminated unnecessary expenditure at the planning and monitoring stage. Economic aspects linked to health repercussions, particularly long-term risks, are not easy to quantify without a correct ex post evaluation.

Input and process of HIA

Input

Following the agricultural firm's request and the doubts arising about the wet zone's possible impacts on population health, a public health professor was commissioned to produce a formal proposal, following in-depth study of the problem and its context. While there was no specific awareness that an HIA-related activity was being undertaken, the City Council wanted to be supported by objective, scientific data in the event that their decision was criticized or attacked by political or community opposition (for this reason no screening process has been performed). The public health professor proposed an HIA activity and asked the City Council to form an ad hoc commission.

Initially the commission comprised a mayoral delegate and two experts: an entomologist and a public health professor. This was expanded to include an epidemiologist and delegates of the agricultural firm and from the population. The commission nominated a steering group involving the mayoral delegate, the three experts and the director of the agricultural firm proposing the project.

Process

The steering group's tasks involved scoping and reporting: meeting three times during the year to define the action plan and task for each component and, at the end, to discuss results and prepare the final report.

The commission was subdivided into groups which involved at least one expert and other stakeholders (farmers, citizens, managers of the proposed construction firm, ecologists and hunters involved in area management). The sub-commissions' tasks generally related to the assessment stage: participants evaluated the topics related directly to their specific competencies.

Briefly, the three experts carried out the evaluation and assessment process through individual analysis, supported by collective discussions. These experts reported results to the Commission from time to time. At the end of the process, the Mayor received four reports: one from each expert and one prepared by the whole Commission. The individual reports were totally bound to their own competencies, based on evaluations focusing on specific aspects (entomology, health and environment). The final report delivered by the Commission tried to interpret the assessment results from different perspectives, including the medical definition of health and broader socioeconomic determinants.

During the assessment phase different tools and methodologies were employed, including:

- literature research
- focus groups
- on-the-spot investigations
- entomological sampling
- water sampling
- agricultural product sampling (olive trees, grapes)
- bacteriological and chemical analysis
- life-quality evaluation with psychometric tools
- interviews
- retrospective epidemiological survey
- entomological analysis
- comparison with similar cases.

The Commission also decided to use collateral plant engineering, and hydrodynamic, botanic and zoological surveys performed by technicians contacted ad hoc. A specific deadline for presenting HIA results was never set up but the formal process concluded in one year.

Following the previous discussion it should be clear that the Mayor took the decision to ask for expert advice in order to avoid problems with the community. Nevertheless the mayoral delegate had a secondary role in the Commission, almost always acting as a facilitator between experts and community stakeholders. The HIA activity was led by the public health professor who had recognized the need for a more in-depth intervention – an HIA which took account of not only the scientific evidence but also the opinions, experiences and expectations of the population.

Community involvement was strong from the beginning. Apart from direct involvement in the work of the Commission, the potentially affected population attended several meetings during the HIA and their opinions were given great consideration. Moreover, the community was constantly informed about the consequences and impacts of the project, and how to control the collateral effects. At the end of the process the City Council gathered in a public assembly at which the Commission's experts presented the final report to the community. This community involvement most likely favoured the fact that both decisions and community dynamics proceeded in parallel with the HIA activity process.

From the beginning, politicians have expressed their positive opinion of the HIA activity; indeed some of them were particularly involved. This did not influence the Commission's work as the elected politicians did not intervene either in favour or against the HIA, neither did they try to influence the stakeholders or the experts. They were privileged witnesses, motivated to push the Commission towards achieving the best possible results for health and economics.

HIA is not a legal requirement in Italy; here the need to solve a community's problem triggered a good practice. Only the first expert contacted was aware of the need to carry out an HIA activity and it is not by chance that this was promoted by a professor of public health, with a significant background in evaluation processes.

All the interviewees agreed that politicians, the community and all the other stakeholders brought irreplaceable contributions to the decision, never competing but always trying to bring their best experiences and competencies to maximize the efficacy of the process and reach the best resolution. There is no clear difference between what was stated by the Mayor and the agricultural firm delegate.

The decision was reached according to the HIA results, as discussed with all the stakeholders. The creation of the wet zone has been planned to run concurrently with the continuous monitoring of environmental and health changes.

Conclusion

Although implemented in a very local setting, the HIA activity produced several results. We hope that this experience will change the approach on the political level (even in a small local setting) to pending decisions, taking into account that each policy has an influence on health that should be considered with proper scientific tools. All the interviewees, from many different points of view, underscored its effectiveness in:

- enabling more thorough deliberations about whether to permit the wet zone;

- increasing community empowerment;

- focusing attention on populations at major levels of risk and taking guaranteed measures (e.g. monitoring and controlled biological parameters but also health indicators) in order to maintain and improve current environmental and health conditions. Monitoring systems were put into action before the damp zone construction, and are carried out at fixed intervals.

It seems that an HIA's effectiveness is influenced positively by the leadership of a well-trained expert who is able to give the HIA direction; continuous involvement of the community; and politicians who facilitate the process but never pressure for one specific decision. However, we should emphasize that the health aims addressed initially by the HIA activity have been the least evaluated for effectiveness: the wet zone is very new and planning of an ex post evaluation study was missed.

This localized experience can bring some considerations to the Italian context, where HIA is very far from being a decision-making tool. Decision-making can be pushed towards an HIA culture with small but effective examples, by working together rather than competing with the population. Moreover, public health has the duty to stimulate this process and to manage the possible criticisms of HIA regarding stakeholder participation and the different aims of science and politics.

Case study 3

A local-level HIA in the transport sector: following legal requirements in Lithuania

Marius Strička, Ingrida Zurlytė and Vilius Grabauskas

Introduction

In Lithuania, the law regulates the assessment of planned economic activities. The impact assessment for proposed economic activities is described in the environmental impact assessment (EIA) of the Planned Economic Activity Act. A strategic plan for any planned economic development must also provide for assessment of the environmental impacts, including economic, health, social and cultural. Such an assessment must cover the entire area in which the plan may be expected to have any impact. In 2004, obligatory health impact assessment (HIA) was introduced for planned economic development where there is a significant potential for negative impacts.

A typical HIA case study was chosen, in which all formal procedures were followed and fulfilled. Reconstruction of the southern railways in the Klaipeda National Seaport will have a significant health impact on populations living in neighbouring areas and in the city of Klaipeda: the reconstruction activities are large-scale and economic activities will double after full implementation in 2015. Residents living in the neighbourhood nearest to the seaport and its railways are already affected negatively by the impacts from the economic activities in the region. The primary health determinants are noise, vibration and pollution from carbon monoxide and solid particulates.

This HIA was effective, but with limitations, since the reconstruction plan was not going to be dropped and only minor modifications to the reconstruction of the southern railways in the Klaipeda National Seaport would be possible.

The study is based on four interviews with participants. The experts represent all the interest groups involved in HIA processes (the client, a representative of the Klaipeda National Seaport and two representatives of the HIA providers) and decisions-makers (a representative of the Public Health Centre responsible for HIA approval). The affected community's representative was not involved in the study, as their role in the process is rather passive. The public was informed about HIA screening results and the report. Local community representatives expressed their willingness for explicit discussions about the report's results but the HIA provider was not aware of any further actions. Public opinion was included indirectly in the HIA report through a local community survey. The HIA documentation for the proposed project has also been analysed.

This chapter begins with a detailed background of the political context of HIA in Lithuania. This is followed by a brief context for the HIA itself, describing the current status of the affected area and processes that were introduced prior to the HIA. A detailed description of the HIA case study details the methods, actors and relationship to the decision-making process. Focus on the HIA's impact clarifies the extent to which it could be judged to be an effective approach – participants felt that the approach had been successful, and these dimensions are discussed in detail. The chapter concludes with a discussion of the processes put in place, and additional factors or inputs which may account for any strengths and weaknesses.

HIA in Lithuania

HIA started in Lithuania in 2004, when the Ministry of Health approved two legal acts, foreseen in the Law on Public Health Care (LR Seimas, 2002) as the supplements EIA (Lietuvos Respublikos, 2004a, 2004b). Lithuania has only a few strategic HIAs, the majority of which are strongly enforced environmental health impact assessments for planned economic activities and development.

HIA is a compulsory procedure for the EIA of planned economic activities if there are significant potential negative impacts, and in the development of territory and construction planning documents. All cases for the compulsory HIA are presented in the HIA cases list under the legislation of EIA for planned economic activities. An HIA has to be carried out if, during economic activity, any negative factors (chemical, biological, socioeconomic, or ergonomic) may directly or indirectly affect the health of the community.

The scientific literature contains some debate about Lithuanian HIA's status as a distinct legal procedure, performed separately from EIA (Ragulskyte-Markoviene & Marcijonas, 2006). The main argument is that this is an outcome of legal over-regulation. In contrast, public health professionals favour the separation of HIA and EIA processes as a stand-alone HIA tends to yield more in-depth analyses of health impacts. It is understood that an EIA of planned economic activity will include an explicit HIA too. However, if planned economic activity is not subject to an EIA, it has to pass the screening procedure for the HIA.

It is also necessary to add that Lithuania has a different political environment and level of community participation, inherited from the Soviet system. Generally speaking, in comparison with older European Union (EU) Member States, community participation levels in decision-making processes are very low and poorly coordinated. In a transitional country, Lithuanian politicians usually prioritize economic benefits rather than health.

A number of institutions (11 public agencies, 9 private companies) were licensed to provide HIA in the State Public Health Service under the Ministry of Health in 2006. HIA providers must include experts with a public health background in the team. EIA providers have no such formal requirement and therefore these may be conducted by private or public companies, as well as directly employed individuals.

The HIA process is much more formalized; as stated above, each planned economic activity during an EIA process is screened for its possible negative health impacts. The State Public Health Service or Regional Public Health Centres are the only institutions allowed to conduct the screening process according to HIA for the planned economic activity or development. An HIA analysis is obligatory if the possible negative health impacts of the proposed economic activity are significant. Only licensed providers are eligible to perform HIAs. It is a formal requirement that the results of a completed HIA are presented in the local print media. The State Public Health Service or Regional Public Health Centres (institutions which provide EIA and HIA screening) are required to assess the expertise of the public health safety levels in an HIA report and either accept or reject it. After formal approval, the proposed economic activity may proceed.

Background to the HIA

Klaipeda National Seaport is located in the western part of Klaipeda city. The seaport's adjoining area contains residential properties with 4069 inhabitants, a kindergarten, a school for children with hearing impairments, a youth centre and several private companies.

The seaport and residential areas are separated by a four-lane road and (twin-track) railways parallel to the road are in seaport territory, separated by a concrete wall. Rail and road transport traffic is very intensive as there are two loading companies at opposite sides of the residential properties.

Local residents complained to Klaipeda Regional Public Health Centre about excessive noise (especially at night) caused by loading works in the seaport and heavy transport crossing the residential area. Noise level measurements of the adjacent area reported increased noise levels (1–10 dBA in the daytime; 10–17 dBA at night). Noise reduction measures were insufficient and sometimes even worsened the situation. Heavy transport traverses the city centre and densely populated urban areas as there is no other route from the seaport. Local residents also requested a measurement of air pollution in the area. Air pollution from solid particulates was almost double the maximum allowed level.

According to the general plan approved by Klaipeda City Municipal Council in 2000, reconstruction of the southern part of Klaipeda National Seaport Railways will be conducted from 2008 to 2015. During the first phase of the project, seaport territory will be expanded to the south-east and a twin-track railway will be constructed. Due to planned construction, the current Nemuno Road will be moved 17 m towards the residential area. Commercial and residential buildings and trees within a new 100 m sanitary zone will be demolished.

During the second phase of the project, nine railway platforms were to be built. Adjacent housing would have been impacted by increased noise levels and construction of four of the nine has been stopped. The number of trains through the reconstructed railway will increase from 4 to 5 trips in 2005 to 12 trips in 2015. Each train has approximately 50 wagons. A cargo terminal for the wagons is planned for the third phase of the project. The marginal planned cargo terminal area will be 30 m to 40 m from residential housing. Planned traffic from the seaport will be 80% railway traffic and 20% road traffic.

Klaipeda Regional Public Health Centre performed the HIA screening of the Klaipeda Seaport Railways Reconstruction Project in August 2004. Measurements of noise and air pollution were taken in the project's affected areas and hygienic examinations were conducted in selected houses adjacent to the seaport and railway. Following the HIA screening results, in-depth HIA analysis was required for the proposed project. The Klaipeda National Seaport Railway Reconstruction Project developers subcontracted HIA analysis to the State Environmental Health Centre, licensed for HIA examination under the Ministry of Health.

The HIA process

Klaipeda Regional Public Health Centre oversaw the HIA of the Southern Railway Reconstruction at Klaipeda National Seaport proposal. The State Environmental Health Centre was subcontracted as an independent HIA provider by Pramprojektas, the company responsible for the initial planning and development of the reconstruction project. Pramprojektas made estimates for the HIA and agreed the timetable for the process. Serving as the main contractor for the HIA team, this company supervised all communications with the client and the overall HIA process. A strict timetable was imposed to ensure that the technical railway plans and legal procedures such as the EIA and HIA would be provided before the final call for EU structural funds. All assessments had to be presented prior to the project's submission to the EU fund office. The initial time scale for the HIA was six months from the date of the agreed assignment.

The HIA was informed by the definition from the Gothenburg consensus (European Centre for Health Policy, 1999) and as described in HIA methodological guidelines. All formal HIA stages such as screening, scoping, appraisal and assessment, recommendations, monitoring, and evaluation were ensured in this process.

In collaboration with the Faculty of Health Science at Klaipeda University, the HIA team of experts completed interviews with residents living in the project's affected area in December 2005. The aim of the survey was to analyse community knowledge about the proposed railway reconstruction project, household satisfaction with living conditions, sources of noise and air pollution, and their impacts on quality of life.

Almost two-thirds of the population involved in the study had never heard about the proposed railway reconstruction. Those who were familiar with the project reported that they had read about it in the local newspaper or received information from their neighbours. A few respondents received information about the railway reconstruction from the municipality stakeholders.

Only half of the respondents were satisfied with their living conditions. More than half stated that, if possible, they would be happy to move from this area. The team recorded positive health effects of the proposed project as railway reconstruction and expansion of the seaport sanitary zone will require sections of housing to be demolished and inhabitants accommodated in new housing. Noise, vibration and air pollution were the main health concerns reported by the households in the affected area. Two-thirds of the households were affected by excessive noise, especially at night. The main sources of noise were rail transport and heavy road transport. Almost half of the respondents also reported that they were disturbed by the docking activities and metalworking.

This population survey proved the findings on noise and air pollution produced during the HIA screening process.

The HIA expert team also initiated an in-depth prognosis of the adverse effects of noise caused by heavy transport during and after railway reconstruction. This indicated that noise levels in most parts of the affected area will increase when the project is implemented. This increase will be associated with negative impacts on health, especially sleeping disturbances. This analysis also indicated that during the last stage of the railway reconstruction, the wagon yard will be built 30 m to 40 m from houses and have a high negative impact on inhabitants' health. Initially, this wagon yard was not presented in the technical project plan and the EIA as the technical part of this project is to be developed during the later stages.

The HIA expert team also analysed road traffic changes (primarily heavy transportation) following the rail reconstruction and improved seaport loading capacities. This is a very significant problem, not only for the inhabitants living near the seaport but also for major parts of Klaipeda.

During the HIA process, national regulations on environmental protection relating to the railway reconstruction and Klaipeda National Seaport activities were analysed for their possible impacts on health. HIA experts also organized study visits to the project site, and held round-table discussions with the project developers' team and the Klaipeda National Seaport administration.

In accordance with HIA methodology regulated by the Ministry of Health, the results of the HIA analysis were presented in the local newspaper. According to the law, each member of the community is informed (through the media) about the HIA report and required to present their opinions and suggestions within 10 days of the report's presentation in the newspaper. The HIA expert team received no comments from the community in response to the analysis.

Effectiveness of the HIA

All parties who participated in the HIA had similar views on the assessment's aims to evaluate major health determinants and propose changes that would help to minimize or prevent negative impacts on community health. There were no alternatives for the proposed technical plans. The HIA experts limited their recommendations to the small number of improvements that were approved during the HIA analysis stage. The HIA prognostic evaluation found that noise levels would increase after the project's implementation. The developers reacted immediately to this finding and offered to build a high-quality acoustic shield on the railway nearest to the neighbouring households. Also the municipality plans to build a crossroad from the city's suburbs to the seaport in response to the HIA's findings on heavy goods vehicles.

The decision-makers for the proposed technical project are not the developers (the HIA client) but rather Klaipeda Regional Public Health Centre which initiated the HIA. The proposed changes to the project will be implemented in large part, as the law strictly regulates the HIA process and requirements. Klaipeda Regional Public Health Centre was also responsible for the HIA analysis approval and took a very firm position during this stage. Although it took part in the HIA, it has dealt primarily with public concerns and all the health impacts of the proposed project will reflect the quality of the Centre's work. The Klaipeda National Seaport administration agreed most of the proposed changes presented by the HIA analysis. Although it may appear a very bureaucratic procedure, the legal basis for the proposed economic activity is heavily supervised. The legal basis of the HIA and the proposed economic activities is the major factor that ensures HIA effectiveness regarding health.

Effectiveness regarding equity has not been analysed in this case study. Although the HIA experts' team analysed the health determinants of vulnerable community groups, no further proposals were presented to stakeholders. The analysis in the HIA was descriptive and this did not lead to concrete proposals.

The HIA had little effectiveness for the community. In accordance with national legislation, HIAs are very bureaucratic and have a limited number of tools to facilitate community participation. Formal meetings between the HIA experts and the client were organized at the HIA team's request but there were no meetings with the community except for interactions during the residents' survey. In contrast, the health complaints presented to the Klaipeda Regional Public Health Centre were included in the HIA assessment and acknowledged appropriately. The HIA analysis report and formal 10-day period for community response were the only tools to secure community participation. There is little evidence of community delegates or representative participation in the decision-making process in Lithuania. In addition, this reconstruction project aims mostly to improve the living conditions of neighbouring residents, and therefore wider community concern is very limited.

The HIA experts noted the organizational effectiveness of the study. Klaipeda University offered support in the provision of the household survey. Also, all experts reported a good atmosphere between themselves, the client and stakeholders.

Factors that facilitated or inhibited effectiveness

All experts participating in the survey stated that, in general, the HIA was effective. Its legal basis was the major factor in this as the HIA and decision-making process is well documented in the methodological HIA guidelines. When they are dedicated to different organizations, separation of the screening, analysis and approval process helps to avoid conflicts of interest. Although the HIA analysis is financed by those proposing the project, they have little or no influence on the approval process.

Health determinants were the major concern of the analysis. The HIA experts and stakeholders represent public health institutions, with a broad understanding of health determinants. The client had little impact on the decision-making process and acted, in this case, mostly as a passive observer and information provider. This may be considered to inhibit the effectiveness of the HIA as the client is almost eliminated from the decision-making process.

The main factor that limited the effectiveness of the HIA is the low community participation level. Community participants usually have their own attitudes and different concerns, which may not be overseen by other stakeholders. HIA legislation leaves communication with the community to the proposed development's planners and this is usually insufficient and irregular.

One of the study's experts also noted that it is quite difficult to make major changes in the technical plans at this stage. Development plans are prepared without the participation of health authorities or the community and therefore not all the proposals which could minimize negative effects or improve health are presented. When a project is presented for an HIA, different options are not presented because of limited timing and decision-making processes. If HIAs began during the planning process, various alternatives could be considered with greater community participation.

All the experts noted timing as an obstacle to HIA effectiveness. In this case study HIA analysis was performed in three weeks – a very short time to provide high-quality, in-depth analysis. Also, there is a limited number of HIA experts in Lithuania, and therefore more intensive training is required, especially at university level.

Conclusion

This typical case study presented a well-developed legal process for an HIA in Lithuania. It is a widely used and effective tool for local projects. Although the process presented health determinants and possible solutions, it required more active participation from the local community. This case has a strong emphasis on environmental health and invites discussion about the overlap between HIA and EIA. Despite this, there is no doubt that the legal requirement for HIA puts health at the top of the agenda when new economic activities are planned.

HIA is a very effective tool on the strategic level when multiple projects or programmes are planned. In Lithuania the HIA legal basis is dedicated to analysing planned economic activities on a single-project level. This HIA was too late to affect decisions on the reconstruction as no alternatives were presented at the initial stage.

It must be acknowledged that public health culture is in its infancy. All levels of government, the media, and all sectors and members of the public have to recognize their role in health improvement.

REFERENCES

European Centre for Health Policy (1999). *Health impact assessment: main concepts and suggested approach. Gothenburg consensus paper.* Copenhagen, WHO Regional Office for Europe (http://www. euro.who.int/document/PAE/Gothenburgpaper.pdf, accessed 13 June 2006).

Lietuvos Respublikos (2004a). Lietuvos Respublikos sveikatos apsaugos ministro 2004 m. liepos 5 d. įsakymas Nr. V-511 „Dėl Lietuvos Respublikos planuojamos ūkinės veiklos poveikio aplinkai vertinimo įstatyme nenumatytų poveikio visuomenės sveikatai vertinimo atvejų ir vertinimo atlikimo taisyklių patvirtinimo" [Order of the Minister of Health of Republic of Lithuania. On adoption of the public health impact assessment cases not foreseen in the Law on Environmental Impact Assessment of Republic of Lithuania and on rules for assessment performace. 5 July 2004 No. V-511].

Lietuvos Respublikos (2004b). Lietuvos Respublikos sveikatos apsaugos ministro 2004 m. liepos 1 d. įsakymas Nr. V-491 „Dėl Poveikio visuomenės sveikatai vertinimo metodinių nurodymų patvirtinimo" [Order of the Ministry of Health of Republic of Lithuania. On adoption of public health impact assessment methodical instructions. 1 July 2004. No. V-491].

LR Seimas (2002). Visuomenės sveikatos priežiūros įsakymas. 2002 m. gegužės 16 d. Nr. IX-886 [Public Health System Law. 16 May 2002. No. IX-886]. Parliament of Republic of Lithuania.

Ragulskytė-Markovienė R, Marcijonas A (2006). Poveikio visuomenės sveikatai ir aplinkai vertinimo santykio problema [Public Health Impact Assessment and Environmental Impact Assessment relationship]. *Sveikatos mokslai [Health Sciences]*, 1–2:108–111.

HIA and intersectoral policy in urban planning: a checklist for health impact screening in Leiden, the Netherlands

Janneke van Reeuwijk-Werkhorst and Loes van Herten

Introduction

Interest in health impact assessment (HIA) in the Netherlands began in the early 1990s. In 1993, the Ministry of Health investigated the feasibility of an HIA system in the country. One recommendation was to start an experimental period of screening of national policy proposals to develop and obtain practical experience with HIA.

The Minister of Health installed an Intersectoral Policy Office (IPO) at the National School of Public Health in 1996 (Roscam Abbing, van Zoest & Varela Put, 1999; Varela Put et al., 2001). This agency commissioned experimental HIAs on national policy proposals, developed HIA methodology and built a network of relevant organizations to practise HIA. After 1999, HIA activities shifted from national towards local level. Interest in intersectoral health policy at the local level has grown since the Public Health Act changed and requires local authorities to take account of health aspects in their administrative decisions (House of Representatives and Senate of the Dutch Parliament, 2002).

The municipality of Leiden, a city in the south-west of the Netherlands, participated in a project to establish tools for intersectoral health policy. The health impact screening (HIS) in Leiden assessed the health impact of a plan for restructuring an industrial area into a residential area, using the checklist for HIS tool (Penris et al., 2004). This case study was selected because interest in HIA on the local level has grown in the last few years. In addition, the case study was well documented due to participation in the national project to develop three tools for intersectoral health policy in municipalities.[4]

The case study was performed when the urban planning was at a stage where there was much attention on health protection, but little or none on health promotion. The HIA led to new consideration of health promotion.

The HIA has had a general effectiveness on health by increasing the consciousness of the decision-makers and by introducing an instrument for reviewing systematically the health aspects of urban planning. It also stimulated new insights, especially regarding lifestyle issues.

No special attention was paid to equity within the HIA itself but the restructuring plan of the area was itself intended to stimulate equity. Its goals were to stimulate the development of houses for people on lower incomes and to improve their existing living conditions, enabling them to stay in the area and even influence their surroundings.

Citizens were involved in the urban planning and had a direct effect on the design of the area. However, the direct effectiveness of community involvement took place at an earlier stage of the urban planning and was not an effect of the HIA.

The Checklist for HIA (Health Effect Screening) was performed during a two-hour session with the urban-planning project group (about 15 people). This meant that it could be executed as a superficial check only, with no in-depth analysis, to see that no health aspects were missed. HIA requires criteria for its use so that it can be introduced clearly as an instrument with a specific place in the policy cycle.

This chapter provides a more detailed background to the policy context of HIA in the Netherlands. This is followed by background information to the HIA, its aims and effectiveness for health, equity and community. Finally, the processes and context are examined as well as the factors that facilitated or inhibited effectiveness of the HIA.

HIA in the Netherlands

The term HIA is not used commonly in the Netherlands; Health Effect Screening is used, a term comparable to HIA Rapid Appraisal as discussed in

---

[4] Both authors were members of the national project team which developed three tools for intersectoral health policy in municipalities, but were not directly involved in the HIA in Leiden.

the Gothenburg consensus (European Centre for Health Policy, 1999; Roscam Abbing, van Zoest & Varela Put, 1999). HIA activities at national level can be divided into two periods.

In the first period (1996–2003), most HIAs were produced or coordinated by the IPO, installed in 1996. Both the Ministry of Health and the IPO made efforts to screen the policies of other ministries for impacts on health. This was intended to be a main activity of the Ministry of Health, with technical support from the IPO. In practice IPO played a major role – producing or coordinating 24 HIAs until 2004. Most HIAs were performed during 1996 to 1999.

In the second period (from 2003) the Ministry of Health stopped funding the IPO. The National Institute for Public Health and the Environment (RIVM) took over some of its functions, including research and networking, e.g. organization of discussion meetings to address HIS and related topics. Until 2006, a budget was available to maintain intersectoral policy in the work of the RIVM.

On the local level, activities are divided into two types of HIA. The first is the HIS methodology for Cities and Environment and is initiated by the Ministry of Housing, Spatial Planning and the Environment and the Ministry of Health. From 1997 to 2003 HIS for Cities and Environment projects were conducted in 25 cities. The other HIA is initiated by the Netherlands Association of Municipal Health Services and the Association of Netherlands Municipalities, and is part of intersectoral health policy at a local level.

There has been greater attention on intersectoral health policy since changes to the Public Health Act required local authorities to take account of health aspects in their administrative decisions (House of Representatives and Senate of the Dutch Parliament, 2002). This aimed to help decision-makers identify and assess health consequences and should raise awareness at local level of the relationships between health and the physical, social and economic environments.

From 2002 to 2004 the Netherlands Association of Municipal Health Services, the National School of Public Health, the RIVM and the Netherlands Organisation for Applied Scientific Research (TNO) worked together on a project to deliver three tools for intersectoral health policy in municipalities (van Reeuwijk-Werkhorst et al., 2005a & 2005b). This was initiated and financed by the steering committee of the National Contract for Public Health. One of these tools was the Checklist for HIS. The National Institute for Health Promotion and Disease Prevention supports municipalities that are implementing intersectoral health policy.

HIS in Leiden

In Leiden, the second type of HIA was performed as the municipality wished to develop an integrated health policy as part of the project to develop three tools for intersectoral health policy in municipalities. The national project team was drawn from the National Association of Municipal Health Services, the Netherlands School of Public & Occupational Health, the National Institute for Public Health and the Environment (RIVM) and the TNO.

The lead agency in Leiden was the local project team which can be seen as a governmental agency as it comprised civil servants from the municipality and municipal health service employees. The municipal officer responsible for public health policy in Leiden was politically accountable (van Herten et al., 2003). The Checklist for HIS (see Appendix) was applied from 2002 to 2003. There was no additional budget available at the local level, and participants viewed it as part of their daily activities (van Herten et al., 2003). The following HIA stages were used: screening, scoping, appraisal and reporting to inform decision-makers. The appraisal phase can be compared to the rapid appraisal.

The Checklist for HIS was used in a local plan to improve a residential and industrial urban area of approximately five hectares. The area had an over-representation of people on lower incomes. Leiden municipality and a local housing association wanted to create an area with transgenerational housing – housing that is durable, appropriate to different stages of life and stimulates social cohesion. In an area that would be 40% car-free they planned approximately 340 rental houses (in different price categories) and 350 building plots. Residents would be involved in controlling the use of the car-free public area (Nieuw Leyden, 2005).

The project group had to deal with the following health-related problems:

- polluted soil which required decontamination;
- gas distribution station which precluded building;
- high voltage cabling, which precluded building;
- proximity of motorway produced noise and air pollution, blocked entrance to green fields at the other side of the street;
- sewage pumping station.

Table CS4.1 *Actors in the Leiden HIA*

Function	Organization
Process leader	Netherlands School of Public & Occupational Health
Civil servant, initiator of HIA	Municipality of Leiden, Department of Welfare and Health Policy
Civil servant, project leader of urban planning	Municipality of Leiden, Department of Housing
Municipal health officer, adviser	Municipal health services in Leiden
Multidisciplinary project group of the urban planning	Municipality of Leiden, different departments
Municipal officer, Housing, Care and Welfare, Leiden North	Municipality of Leiden
Population of District North, interactive policy process	Inhabitants of Leiden

Source: Based on Herten van, et al. (2003) and interviews, March and April 2006.

The project group formulated the following objectives for the new residential area:

- retain historical buildings;
- connect (in an ecological way) the new residential area with a green area that lies to the north, across the main road;
- impose low speed limit (30 km zone);
- decrease parking spaces (to increase living space) and build garages under houses (approx 400);
- stimulate people to stay in the area (own house development);
- improve living conditions for lower-income residents;
- improve population mix by including more expensive houses.

Those who participated in the HIA are shown in Table CS4.1. The population of District North was involved at an earlier stage of the urban planning in 1998.

Time frame of urban planning

The time frame of the urban planning is shown in Table CS4.2. The HIA was performed during 2002 and 2003.

Interviewees

In March and April 2006 interviews were held with the civil servant who initiated the HIA, the civil servant who was the project leader of urban planning and the adviser working in municipal health services in Leiden.

Table CS4.2 *Time frame of urban planning in Leiden*

1997	First plans for restructuring the northern area in Leiden
1998	Active participation of Leiden inhabitants
2001	Start project group. Objectives defined
2002	State aid (financial)
2002–2003	Checklist for HIS executed
2004	Start preparation phase
2005	City Council approves project
2006	Start building
2009	Finalization

Source: Based on Nieuw Leyden (2005) and interviews, March and April 2006.

Also, we spoke with the process leader from the Netherlands School of Public & Occupational Health who was involved in this project. She gave us relevant process and contextual information on performing the HIA. We also used our own experience as members of the national project team on intersectoral health policy.

Aims of the HIA

The municipality of Leiden wanted to develop an integrated health policy and therefore participated in a project to establish tools for intersectoral health policy. The civil servant from the welfare and health policy department selected a case for the HIA: restructuring an industrial and residential area into a residential area.

One of the interviewees indicated that the trigger to perform an HIA was the desire to gain experience of intersectoral health policy and incorporate it within the local health plan of the municipality. Also he was searching for an instrument to structure the local health plan that municipalities in the Netherlands are obliged to formulate and execute every four years. The municipal officer responsible for public health policy in Leiden "is dedicated to health policy" which stimulated the use of HIA.

Initially, the added value of the HIA was not clear to the project leader of the urban planning:

> At the start of the development plan, health aspects were already taken into account, because industry elements triggered this. I was afraid that the HIA should delay the urban planning. We had already formulated our starting-points and objectives. But I agreed upon the HIA in order to check if we were taking all health elements into account.

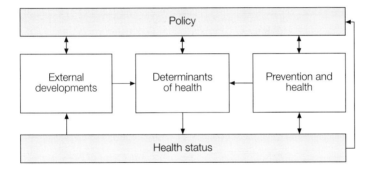

Figure CS4.1 *VTV-model of health*

Dimensions of effectiveness

Health effectiveness

A wide range of factors determine the health of a population. The Checklist for HIS is based on the Centre for Public Health Broadcasting (VTV) health concept. This VTV-model[5] explains health as a result of a multi-causal process with different determinants (Figure CS4.1). The model is based on Lalonde's model (Lalonde, 1974) in which the health status of the population is influenced by biological factors, lifestyle factors, physical and social environment, and health care services, including prevention. This model is often used as the basis for the design and study of health policies in the Netherlands.

The HIA's report made recommendations for further investigations into the problems of air pollution, noxious smells, noise, high-voltage infrastructure and ventilation of garages. It also recommended the preparation of a plan to stimulate social cohesion in the area. The HIA's results were summarized in the local health plan. One respondent stated that "the HIA stimulated consciousness and new insights. HIA led to a check that all elements were included in the plans. Especially lifestyle issues delivered new insights."

None of the three respondents was definitely sure that the decision-making was influenced directly by the HIA. Health aspects in relation to the environment (e.g. air and soil pollution) were taken into account at an early stage of the urban planning. The focus was on health protection. All three interviewees indicated that this was obvious because of the industrial history of the area. Nevertheless, the HIA revealed new insights on lifestyle factors principally, especially the opportunities to stimulate physical activity. These factors are considered to be health promoting.

[5] http://www.rivm.nl/vtv/object_document/o5423n30044.html Accessed 4 September 2006.

Two of the three interviewees indicated that the HIA had a general effect on health by increasing the consciousness of decision-makers and by introducing an instrument for systematic review of the health aspects of urban planning. As a result of the HIA, the City Council has identified intersectoral health policy as one of the two priorities for local health policy 2003–2006 "to stimulate awareness for health-related effects of policy proposals" (Boelens & Bats, 2003). However, not all policy proposals will be screened for health impacts – only those with links to environment and health, or physical environment (defined as living, care and well-being) and health.

One of the respondents mentioned that the Checklist for HIS will be used in another urban planning project in Leiden. Furthermore, from time to time all civil servants will be reminded of the need to be aware of the health-related effects of existing and new policies (van Leeuwen, 2005).

Equity effectiveness

In the HIA itself no special attention was paid to equity. One interviewee explained that the restructuring plan in itself intended to stimulate equity. In 1996 the municipality of Leiden started working with '*Wijk Ontwikkelings Plannen (WOP)*' or area development plans. These aim to connect the physical, economic and social aspects of urban life. One of the basic principles of the area development plan for Leiden-North is to stimulate social cohesion and give people with lower incomes the opportunity to buy a house. In the current population of the area there is an over-representation of lower income groups. One of the objectives of the restructuring plan was to introduce more expensive houses and to stimulate own house development, in order to encourage people to stay in the area, especially when they start to earn more money and intend to leave the area. Another objective of the plan was to improve the living surroundings for people with lower incomes.

Community effectiveness

Two interviewees mentioned the importance of the interactive process between citizens and municipality. This community involvement in urban planning increased the attention on health. Citizens want a healthy living environment and their involvement was seen as a positive impulse for urban planning. However, this was not an effect of the HIA as it took place at an earlier stage of the urban planning.

With 118 000 inhabitants Leiden is considered a big city in the Netherlands. The Dutch Government has a special policy for increasing citizens' quality of life by integrating physical, economic and social aspects of city life –

Grotestedenbeleid. Citizens were involved from the very beginning of the project (e.g. theatre sessions, interviews and visualization of their ideas), having a direct influence on the design of the area such as playgrounds for children, open spaces rather then parking spaces. Citizens were positive about this involvement which had positive effects on their relationships with civil servants from the municipality. However, when definite plans were decided they were only passively involved – informed about results and ideas, but not consulted again.

Other dimensions of effectiveness

The civil servant who had initiated the HIA changed jobs. This was considered to be important in disrupting continuity and therefore affecting administrative effectiveness. However, the municipality report on local health policy 2003–2006 stated that "the HIA seems to be a useful instrument" and they are considering using this tool in another comparable situation in Leiden (van Leeuwen, 2005).

Process, input and context of HIA

Process

The Checklist for HIA was under construction at the time it was used as Leiden took part in a pilot to develop its use in municipalities. It took some time to obtain formal permission for participation in the pilot project. One interviewee stated that "the decision-makers doubted the need and usefulness of HIA."

In this case study the Checklist for HIA was performed during a two-hour session with the urban planning project group (about 15 people). The group was multidisciplinary and consisted of a project assistant, traffic planner, environmental expert, air, soil and water specialists, town and country planners, and members of the HIA local project team. The time constraint meant that the Checklist for HIA could be executed only superficially, with no in-depth analysis. It was used literally as a means of checking to see that no health aspects were missed and to confirm that the right actions were taken. When this was completed, the municipal health representative and the civil servant for welfare and health policy worked out the determinants of health related to the problems of the area. Recommendations were formulated and reported to the City Council (van Herten et al., 2003; Municipal Health Services South-Holland North, 2003).

All three interviewees perceived the timing of the HIA to be "too late" in the policy process. The focus was health protection rather than on both health protection and health promotion. HIA undertaken at an earlier stage could take account of both health and environmental issues, such as air and soil pollution.

Two respondents advised integrating or linking the instruments for environmental impact assessment (EIA) and HIA, because these instruments are closely related.

Input and context

It was suggested that the results of the HIA could be used as a tool for communicating with citizens, as they demonstrate that the municipality takes health issues seriously. This could improve citizens' confidence in health issues.

Civil servants perceive instruments like the Checklist for HIA as an extra workload to the existing rules and instruments within the organization. This requires a clear introduction of the applications of HIA and its place in the policy cycle. It is not feasible to check every plan for its consequences on health but criteria for the use of HIA could be helpful in selecting relevant plans (e.g. schools, living areas). The benefits of the HIA should be pointed out quickly to potential users although this is hindered by the difficulty of quantifying the results.

Conclusion

In analysing the case study a distinction can be made between HIA's effectiveness for two different goals of HIA: health protection and health promotion. The case study was performed when urban planning was at a stage when the focus was on health protection (e.g. polluted soil, air pollution) with little or no attention to health promotion (e.g. physical activity). The HIA did lead to new thoughts about health promotion.

In this case, an HIA could have been carried out at two different stages of the urban planning. Initially it required an HIA focused on health protection but at a later stage it required a focus on health promotion. This could be one of the recommendations for HIA practitioners promoting and embedding HIA in organizations.

The findings of this case study led to other conclusions and recommendations detailed below.

Introduce clearly the instrument of HIA and its place in the policy cycle

HIA can be perceived as time-consuming, increasing the workload of potential users and competing with organizations' existing rules and instruments.

Clear introduction of the HIA instrument, with special attention to its benefits for potential users as well as its place in the policy cycle, could address these concerns and contribute to more extensive use of this instrument.

Outline criteria for use

It is not feasible to check every plan for its consequences on health. HIA is suggested for use for plans or buildings where many people are involved, e.g. schools, residential areas.

Combine or integrate HIA with other health-related instruments

HIA competes with other closely related health instruments, e.g. EIA. It can be efficient to combine or integrate with (parts of) these instruments.

Communicate HIA results to citizens

This case study shows that community involvement in urban planning has a positive effect on the relationship with municipal civil servants by improving citizens' confidence in the municipality's concern for health. This confidence could be strengthened by informing citizens about the results of an HIA.

REFERENCES

Boelens B, Bats H (2003). *Nota Lokaal Gezondheidsbeleid 2003–2006. Een kaderstelling voor het gemeentelijk gezondheidsbeleid [Local health policy 2003–2006]*. Leiden, B&W [Board of Mayor and Aldermen] (Nr. 03.0715/30-06-2003).

European Centre for Health Policy (1999). *Health impact assessment: main concepts and suggested approach. Gothenburg consensus paper*. Brussels, WHO Regional Office for Europe (http://www.euro.who.int/document/PAE/Gothenburgpaper.pdf, accessed 13 June 2006).

Herten LM van, et al. (2003). *Instrumenten voor facetbeleid: projectverslag [Report on instruments for integrated local health policy]*. Leiden/Bilthoven, TNO Preventie en Gezondheid, RIVM, NSPOH, GGD Nederland.

House of Representatives and Senate of the Dutch Parliament (2002). *House of Representatives and Senate of the Dutch Parliament, 2001–2002, Act of 13th July 2002 to amend the Public Health Act (Wcpv)*. The Hague, Staatsblad 468.

Lalonde M (1974). *A new perspective on the health of Canadians: a working document*. Ottawa, Government of Canada.

Leeuwen A van (2005). *Stand van zaken notitie Lokaal Gezondheidsbeleid 2003–2006 [Update of local health policy 2003–2006]*. Leiden, B&W [Board of Mayor and Aldermen] (Nr. 05.0476 d.d.).

Municipal Health Services South-Holland North (2003). Letter from Municipal Health Services South-Holland North (GGD Zuid-Holland Noord) to the Board of Mayor and Aldermen (het College van B&W). Advies n.a.v. pilot checklist GES project EWR/Slachthuis [Advice regarding pilot project HIS in Leiden]. Leiden, 26 August 2003.

Nieuw Leyden (2005). *Uitvoeringsdocument EWR+/Slachthuisterrein [Realisation document industrial area, including slaughterhouse]*. Municipality of Leiden, 8 March 2005 (http://www.

keicentrum.nl/view.cfm?page_id=1893&item_type=nieuws&item_id=526, accessed 4 September 2006; http://www.stedplan.nl/index.php?reload=1&referer=, accessed 4 September 2006; http://www.leiden.nl/dspage.asp?objectid=31989&sessionid=1CWRZ5zCSvofBaqys 3l54qVxDU@t5K78Ld!zmM!6Az1JIodrhoUhCp3M4aGxJh@O, accessed 4 September 2006; http://www.nieuwleyden.nl, accessed 4 September 2006).

Penris M, et al. (2004). *Handboek checklist gezondheidseffectscreening [Handbook checklist health impact screening]*. Bilthoven/Leiden/Utrecht, RIVM/NSPOH/TNO/GGD-Nederland.

Reeuwijk-Werkhorst J van, et al. (2005a). Methoden voor integraal gezondheidsbeleid. Ontwikkeling en toepassing in gemeenten [Development and assessment of methods for integrated local health policy]. *TSG Tijdschrift voor gezondheidswetenschappen*, 83(7):418–424.

Reeuwijk-Werkhorst J van, et al. (2005b). Development and assessment of tools for intersectoral local health policy in the Netherlands (Abstract). *Italian Journal of Public Health*, 2(2): suppl.1.

Roscam Abbing EW, Zoest FF van, Varela Put G (1999). Health impact assessment and intersectoral policy at national level in the Netherlands. In: *Health impact assessment – from theory to practice*. Report on the WHO Regional Office for Europe and the Nordic School of Public Health Leo Kaprio Workshop. Gothenburg: 28–30 October 1999.

RVZ: Council for Public Health and Health Care (2000a). *Gezond zonder zorg [Healthy without care]*. Zoetermeer, RVZ: Council for Public Health and Health Care.

RVZ: Council for Public Health and Health Care (2000b). *Gezond zonder zorg: achtergrondstudies [Healthy without care: background studies]*. Zoetermeer, RVZ: Council for Public Health and Health Care.

Varela Put G, et al. (2001). *Experience with HIA at national policy level in the Netherlands*. Copenhagen and Brussels, European Centre for Health Policy (Policy Learning Curve Series, No. 4, September).

Appendix

The Checklist for HIS is a practical tool used to evaluate specific policy proposals with regard to their relevance to health and their potential health effects. The goal is to provide input on health issues for areas other than health. There are three distinct stages:

1 screening of health-relevant policy plans (case-finding);
2 analysis and description of potential health impact (HIA);
3 influencing planned policies (intersectoral policy).

The Checklist for HIS for local use is a questionnaire in three parts:

1 structured questionnaire to gain insight into policy plan, which includes health aspects and target groups;
2 assess health relevance of the policy plan on basis of determinants of health (e.g. lifestyle, environmental factors, social factors, health care);
3 action template to convert results from two into tangible actions.

A city council's air quality action plan: building capacity for HIA in Northern Ireland

Teresa Lavin and Owen Metcalfe

Introduction

HIA is gaining increasing attention in Northern Ireland as a means of influencing public policy in favour of health. *Investing for Health*, the cross-departmental public health strategy, identifies HIA as a key tool to facilitate cross-sectoral action and as a means of promoting health and reducing inequalities (Department of Health, Social Services and Public Safety, 2002).

This case study reviews a comprehensive, prospective HIA which was undertaken on a city Council's draft air quality action plan. The Council was one of the main drivers for the HIA and therefore this is a good example of the added value that HIA can offer in the development of plans or policies. This will be explored with regard to three main areas: (i) bringing a particular health focus to the Air Quality Action Plan (ii) strengthening the involvement of other agencies whose work influences air quality (iii) as a means of engaging with the community.

The information for this case study is based on interviews with six individuals who were involved with the HIA. Three interviewees were members of the management team, responsible for much of the data collection and for overseeing the HIA. The other three were members of the HIA steering group. The steering group included one member of staff from the Institute of Public Health but this individual was not interviewed. Draft and final reports of both the HIA and the Air Quality Action Plan were also reviewed.

Five semi-structured interviews were conducted over a one-month period from March to April 2006. One interview was held with two representatives from the same organization at that organization's request, to expedite the interview process. The questions that formed the basis of the interview were sent out in advance. Interviewees included:

- an environmental health manager and a technical officer for air quality from the City Council;

- the Director of the local Healthy Cities organization;

- a senior engineer from the roads service division of the Northern Ireland Government Department of Regional Development;

- a specialist registrar in Public Health from the regional Health and Social Services Board;

- an environmental officer from the regional integrated public transport company.

An external consultant engaged to conduct the HIA and guide the process was not interviewed; however, the consultant's comments on a draft of this case study have been included. Attempts to interview a community representative/member of the affected population were unsuccessful.

Profiling the HIA

The City Council's draft Air Quality Action Plan was compiled as part of the process of complying with the Government's Air Quality Strategy for England, Scotland, Wales and Northern Ireland, which establishes a series of health-based objectives for eight key air pollutants (Department of the Environment, Transport and the Regions, 2000). The Environment (Northern Ireland) Order 2002 (Office of Public Sector Information, 2002) stipulates that if the levels of one or more of these pollutants are likely to exceed any of the relevant objectives, the District Council is required to designate the location(s) as an Air Quality Management Area (AQMA) and develop an Air Quality Action Plan to reduce the concentration of pollutants. Following the City Council's assessment of air quality conducted in 2003, four areas were designated AQMAs. The next stage in the process was to develop an Air Quality Action Plan (hereafter referred to as the Action Plan) within a one-year time frame commencing in August 2004.

The City Council was aware that measures proposed by other councils during the development of Air Quality Action Plans were not always effective and in some cases could actually contribute to negative impacts. One of the Council respondents said " ... I didn't want us to get it wrong, that we'd end up with actions that were all about roads and road functions and maybe public transport, but in reality weren't actually deliverable".

The City Council had responsibility to develop and implement this Action Plan but, as all four AQMAs border major arterial roads, it was recognized that the main source of air pollution in these areas was road transport, which is outside their remit. This led to interest in working with other organizations that had responsibility in this area, primarily the roads service section of the Department for Regional Development. Although a statutory consultation process would take place, one of the Council respondents expressed a view that " ... we wanted to deliver more than just a consultation ... Air quality is a bit of a dead subject for people and we could send out 300 documents and ask people's views and we won't get any back". Thus there was an interest in exploring ways over and above the statutory consultation process to make the Action Plan as effective as possible.

The identification of HIA as a methodology to assess the potential health impacts of the Action Plan was the result of a combination of factors. HIA is one of the core themes of the current World Health Organization European Healthy Cities Network programme (WHO Regional Office for Europe, 2003). With partner organizations, the local Healthy Cities organization had identified a number of projects suited to an HIA, one of which was the Action Plan. There was already a good working relationship between the City Council and the local Healthy Cities organization. In addition, a number of Council personnel had attended HIA training and were aware of its potential to influence policy and plan development. Also the Regional Health Board was interested in becoming involved with a relevant HIA project. Air quality is of major importance to health and therefore the Public Health Department deemed this HIA to be an appropriate project.

The concept of HIA was understood as being "a combination of procedures, methods and tools by which a policy, programme or project may be judged as to its potential effects on the health of a population, and the distribution of those effects within the population" (European Centre for Health Policy, 1999). The HIA was conducted at the local level, in the four AQMAs referred to earlier. These not only bordered major arterial roads but also were areas of high socioeconomic deprivation.

An external consultant was engaged to conduct the HIA and guide the process using a rapid appraisal tool that she had developed (Ison, 2002). Guidance developed by the Institute of Public Health in Ireland (Doyle, Metcalfe & Devlin, 2003) was also referred to. A broad determinants of health model was assumed at the outset, however those respondents with a remit for health expressed a view that there were different levels of understanding of this model amongst steering group members.

Initial discussions about the HIA began in late 2004; most of the work was conducted in the first six months of 2005. There were five steering group meetings – the last in July 2005. Members of the management team met more frequently as they took responsibility for much of the evidence gathering. Evidence from the literature and a number of consultation events was collated and presented to the steering group in June 2005. A draft of the HIA report was produced in June 2005 and the final report and a summary document were published in May 2006. As stated previously, the HIA was conducted on the draft Action Plan. An early version of the final Action Plan was available in December 2005 and the final report was published in May 2006. It should be noted that HIA interviews took place in March and April 2006, before the final reports had been published. It should also be noted that four of the interviewees were involved with the development of the Action Plan.

Aims and objectives of the HIA

The overall aim of the HIA was to suggest ways of modifying the Action Plan in order to maximize positive, and minimize negative, health impacts. All respondents generally agreed that the HIA was undertaken to bring an added health focus. Some respondents focused on the mitigation aspects, viewing the HIA as a check to ensure that the plan did not influence health negatively in any unforeseen way. Others, mostly from organizations with a specific remit for health, saw additional opportunities to enhance potential positive aspects of the Action Plan.

The HIA was also seen as a way to improve the quality of engagement with the community. A statutory consultation process would take place whether or not the HIA went ahead but it was anticipated that the HIA had the potential to gain community ownership of, and participation in, the process and thus make the Action Plan more effective. In addition, all respondents felt that the community would provide valuable insights that could not be provided by the statutory participants.

There was interest in using the HIA as a means to engage more fully with other agencies, particularly those with responsibility for traffic. As outlined earlier, the Council was responsible for developing and implementing the Action Plan even though it was recognized by all respondents that one of the major causes of air pollution within the AQMAs was road transport. Agencies with a specific remit in this area would be critical to implementation of recommendations around road use and traffic management.

HIA is a relatively new concept in Northern Ireland but one that is gaining increasing interest. There was general recognition that this was a new skill area. Four respondents from organizations which were the main drivers for the HIA indicated that an underlying objective for their involvement was to develop expertise in the use of the HIA methodology.

The Council was one of the main drivers of the HIA, and its aim was " ... about minimizing the detrimental health impacts and improving the positive aspects ... but there were also other issues of inclusiveness and effectiveness of the plan which all came along with the HIA process".

Dimensions of effectiveness

Most respondents pointed out that an assessment of effectiveness was premature, as the process had not reached its conclusion, and made without access to all the facts (the Action Plan had not been published when the interviews took place). However, there was concurrence that overall the HIA had been useful and worthwhile, particularly in raising the profile of health. In the words of one Council representative: " ... there was definitely a change from resistance to believing to accepting – the HIA process and community workshops contributed to that."

All respondents agreed that it was too early to assess effectiveness in terms of outcomes such as air quality improvements over and above what would have been achieved by the Action Plan alone. It was asserted that this is partly because air quality standards typically are assessed in terms of annual means and therefore it will take some time to establish clear trends. Moreover, it was acknowledged that attributing effect to specific causes within the complexity of air quality standards added to the overall challenge.

Health effectiveness

There was concurrence regarding general health effectiveness in terms of increased awareness of health. All respondents felt that this was a particular benefit of the HIA, fulfilling one of its aims – to bring a health focus to the Action Plan. It was felt that, for a number of organizations/agencies involved, the HIA process had brought about greater understanding of the links between the wider determinants of health and air quality. Respondents representing the City Council, Healthy Cities and the Regional Health Board highlighted that one of the most effective ways of getting people to consider health was through the provision of a community health profile, which presented relevant health statistics.

There was less concurrence on whether the strategic objectives relating to health in the Action Plan had been changed as a result of the HIA. One respondent, who was also involved in the development of the Action Plan, expressed the view that this was not necessarily a problem as this already addressed health issues. The HIA process was probably more influential in strengthening rather than changing strategic objectives.

Equity effectiveness

There were mixed responses regarding equity effectiveness: four respondents indicated general effectiveness, two suggested that there was direct effectiveness as a result of the HIA. From the Council's perspective, equity was key to the whole process and its respondents felt that it had influenced the Action Plan. Respondents from other organizations indicated that while there was increased acknowledgment of equity issues, they were less inclined to believe that this had influenced the Action Plan. However, highlighting the impact of socioeconomic status on health was felt to be one way in which equity effectiveness was achieved. In the words of the Health Board representative: "A lot of the measures in the Action Plan would have addressed air quality generally but the HIA highlighted that the health in these areas (the four AQMAs) was worse anyway because of socioeconomic disadvantage."

Community effectiveness

Responses about community effectiveness were mixed: half of the respondents indicated that there was direct effectiveness, the others felt that community interest was acknowledged but did not influence the Action Plan. Responses followed similar patterns for community and equity effectiveness, with the exception of the respondent representing the integrated public transport organization who indicated that there was direct effectiveness with regard to community. Those who reported direct effectiveness identified clear links between suggestions made at the community workshops and actions outlined in the final Action Plan. This was summarized by one of the Council representatives:

> ... the HIA process highlighted a number of community concerns which were fed back to the relevant organizations for further comment and the responses of those organizations which considered these concerns have been included in the final air quality Action Plan.

For other measures of effectiveness, there was a general view that the HIA had impacted positively on working partnerships between different organizations. One respondent felt that this had not been maximized but others saw it as the beginning of a slow sea change that could not be rushed. Overall, it was felt that valuable lessons had been learnt and foundations laid for future work. The importance of this cooperation was summed up by one respondent: "The HIA was a partnership but the whole Air Quality Plan is about partnership".

Factors influencing effectiveness

Process

As stated earlier, four of the interviewees were also involved in the development of the Action Plan and thus had direct knowledge of how this process was developing and the timing of decisions. For those involved in the HIA alone, there appeared to be a general awareness of the deadlines which needed to be met in order to influence the final Action Plan.

Overall, there were positive comments on the methodology and rigour of the HIA process. Respondents indicated that the presence of an external consultant helped to guide the process which contributed to effectiveness. Even the main drivers of the HIA identified an initial lack of clarity about how the HIA would differ from a consultation but the external consultant helped to clarify this.

With regard to the stages of the HIA, one respondent had been involved in the screening process and another knew that it had taken place. Both of these respondents were closely involved with the initiation of the HIA. According to both, it had been agreed in advance to proceed with the HIA and therefore the screening activity was used to highlight the elements that would be included rather than to decide whether or not to proceed. While current methodology indicates that the outcome of screening is to decide whether or not to proceed with an HIA, Northern Ireland has no formal process for selecting proposals for which an HIA should be considered, therefore other reasons are likely to influence this decision. The combination of factors outlined earlier thus provides a useful insight into what is driving the HIA process.

According to the respondents from the Council, initially it was thought that the HIA could best contribute to the consultation element of the Action Plan's development. The scope of the HIA was soon extended as it became clear that it would be of sufficient technical and scientific significance to exist as a separate document.

The management team was responsible for gathering most of the data but all respondents indicated that they contributed data as required. Communities were engaged in a number of different ways using some innovative methods, for example, schoolchildren were asked to express their views on air quality and health through a school art competition.

Most of the respondents were involved in an appraisal workshop and all of those involved indicated that this had been a positive experience. However, two respondents expressed a view that this did not achieve its potential to extract the maximum amount of information as not all groups had professionals with specific skills or training in facilitation.

The external consultant was responsible for writing up the HIA report. Respondents raised two issues relating to this report. Firstly, there appears to have been some debate about the validity or acceptability of different forms of evidence – some steering group members questioned some of the findings. This was explained by one of the Council respondents:

> [Some agencies] would have been looking at some of (the external consultant's) comments and saying well, that's not true and then it would have been pointed out (by the consultant) that this has come out of the workshop and it's been said, therefore it's a valid comment. So, we had a bit of debate on that ... down to a measured agreement on it.

However, another respondent, representing the Healthy Cities organization, felt that the debate was largely unnecessary: "For me, if you employ an independent expert/HIA assessor, then you [should] agree largely with the suggestions made [by that person]."

The second issue related to the length of the final report. While it was generally agreed that this was a comprehensive piece of work, three respondents expressed the view that it was too voluminous to be digested by decision-makers and this detracted from its usability. At the final steering group meeting in July 2005 it was decided to produce a summary report but this was not published until May 2006. Two respondents suggested that the lack of a further meeting and/or a perceived lack of clarity regarding signing off the HIA report may have contributed to this delay. However, the two Council respondents pointed out that key issues were identified quickly after the HIA workshops and presented to decision-makers and, in their opinion, the production of the actual report was not a major factor.

Input

The enthusiasm and resource support from the developers of the proposal on which the HIA was conducted appeared to have been a major factor in driving the process forward. In addition, the HIA process had the potential to meet multiple agendas (as outlined earlier) which was seen as very favourable to obtaining initial approval and funding.

Context

While there is no legislative mandate for HIA in Northern Ireland, two respondents felt that the Investing for Health Strategy was a strong driver for HIA; others expressed a willingness to engage with the process as it was seen as a way to improve the plan. There were mixed views on whether or not health was considered sufficiently at strategic decision-making level. Those from organizations with a health remit were more likely to express the view that it was given insufficient consideration. In general, it was felt that there was a good understanding of health impacts at delivery level but a perceived lack of coordination and communication between the agencies charged with delivery.

There were mixed responses on whether or not the HIA is politically controversial. One respondent felt that while not politically controversial, it is, or has the potential to be, a huge addition to an already heavy workload. Given its non-statutory basis, this may have implications for future willingness to engage with the process.

Conclusion

The interviews were held March–April 2006 when the final Air Quality Action Plan and the summary HIA report were being finalized. This timing may have contributed in part to the respondents' divergence of views on the effectiveness of the HIA. Some of these issues have been resolved by reviewing both documents since publication and returning to interviewees for clarification.

This was a comprehensive HIA funded by the Environment and Heritage Service section of the Department of the Environment and Belfast City Council, which also had a statutory obligation to develop the Air Quality Action Plan. This is an example of the advantages and disadvantages that can occur when the same organization drives both the HIA and the proposal upon which it is based.

One issue warranting further mention is the divergence of views between those involved in the HIA and the development of the Action Plan or the HIA alone. Two respondents were closely involved with both, two were members of both steering groups and two were closely involved with the HIA but not the Action Plan itself. One of the respondents involved in the HIA alone felt that this could make it more difficult to identify precisely the ways in which the

HIA influenced the Action Plan as it would have been a continual process. However, she concluded that the involvement of an external consultant may have contributed positively as it introduced more objectivity into the HIA process. Those involved in both the Action Plan and the HIA largely viewed it as beneficial, according to one of the Council respondents:

> I ran the thing parallel because we knew from early partnership stages with our air quality caps on that it was going to be a tough battle to win hearts and minds and to get to the point of producing this document [with] all these other organizations …
> it was quite timely as we were trying to engender that slow sea change in the other organizations.

REFERENCES

Department of the Environment, Transport and the Regions (2000). *The air quality strategy for England, Scotland, Wales and Northern Ireland*. Norwich, Government Stationery Office.

Department of Health, Social Services and Public Safety (2002). *Investing for health*. Belfast, Department of Health, Social Services and Public Safety.

Doyle C, Metcalfe O, Devlin J (2003). *Health impact assessment: a practical guidance manual*. Dublin, Institute of Public Health in Ireland.

European Centre for Health Policy (1999). *Health impact assessment: main concepts and suggested approach. Gothenburg consensus paper*. Brussels, WHO Regional Office for Europe (http://www.euro.who.int/document/PAE/Gothenburgpaper.pdf, accessed 15 June 2006).

Ison E (2002). *Rapid appraisal tool for health impact assessment: a task-based approach*. Commissioned by the Directors of Public Health of Berkshire, Buckinghamshire, Northamptonshire and Oxfordshire. Supported by the Faculty of Public Health Medicine (http://www.fph.org.uk/policy_communication/downloads/publications/toolkits/Rapid_appraisal_toolkit/Introduction.pdf, accessed 15 June 2006).

Office of Public Sector Information (2002). The Environment (Northern Ireland) Order. Statutory Instrument No. 3153 (N.I.7). Surrey, The Stationery Office (http://www.opsi.gov.uk/si/si2002/uksi_20023153_en.pdf, accessed 15 June 2006).

WHO Regional Office for Europe (2003). *Phase IV (2003–2008) of the WHO Healthy Cities Network in Europe: goals and requirements*. Copenhagen, WHO Regional Office for Europe.

Case study 6

Using intersectoral networks towards the adoption of the Common Agricultural Policy: an HIA on the Food and Nutrition Action Plan in Slovenia

Mojca Gabrijelčič Blenkuš [6] and Nina Scagnetti

Introduction

Food policy has an enormous and complex influence on the health of the inhabitants of any country (Lock, 2004). Slovenia joined the Common Agricultural Policy (CAP) system when joining the European Union (EU), prompting the Ministry of Health of the Republic of Slovenia (MoH) to try to estimate the consequences for the health of Slovenia's population. This was the basic reason for conducting the health impact assessment (HIA) on food and agricultural policies and on the potential effects of Slovenia's accession to the EU. In Slovenia the Gothenburg consensus (European Centre for Health Policy, 1999) definition of HIA is translated as "ocena vplivov na zdravje".

In addition to the twin pillars of food safety and nutrition, the Food and Nutrition Action Plan for Slovenia (FNAP), following WHO first FNAP (WHO 2001), is based also on a third – food security. If established properly this could enable individuals to gain easier access to healthy foods thereby

---

[6] Mojca Gabrijelčič Blenkuš has been engaged as a member of a working group conducting HIA.

reducing the rates of diseases linked to poor nutrition. HIA enabled the integration of this food supply pillar within the FNAP (Ministry of Health of the Republic of Slovenia, 2005), helping to establish intersectoral cooperation on various levels (Gregorič & Fajdiga Turk, 2005). It has also helped to identify joint developmental goals, including agriculture in regional developmental plans, carried out through the established partnership in the north-east region of Pomurje (Buzeti, Buzeti & Belović, 2004).

The intention of this case study is to study how effectively the HIA methodology was used to assess the complex national policies relating to a specific food-policy process. The material in this chapter is based on interviews with key informants, and analysis and interpretation of qualitative data gathered from the interviews.

Profiling the HIA within the national context

The situation of food policy and public health is generally complex. There is strong scientific evidence that food and nutrition are significant factors in the rise of obesity and noncommunicable diseases such as cardiovascular disease sand some cancers, major causes of premature death in Slovenia. Since accession, the national food policy has been influenced significantly by the CAP which is characterized by its support for producers and trade. Despite the emphasis on public health in the Maastricht and Amsterdam Treaties, the EU food and agricultural policies have limited public health implications. At the same time, there is growing public concern about food safety and quality, production methods and environmental contamination. The challenge facing Slovenia was to balance the national concerns of citizens, farmers and the food industry with EU law and public health (Lock et al., 2004b).

The MoH was worried about how the accession, especially changes in agriculture, would affect the health status of Slovenians. Slovenia was undergoing rapid transition prior to EU accession in 2004 (Albreht at al., 2002). The country has several major health problems, which includes one of the highest national rates of suicide and liver cirrhosis in Europe and generally diminished health conditions in the eastern part of the country. The north-east region has the highest mortality rate and the largest agricultural sector of any Slovenian region – 20% of the population is employed in farming or related industries (Šelb & Kravajna, 2000). This part of the country was most likely to be affected by accession (Buzeti, Buzeti & Belović, 2004).

The MoH set out to undertake an HIA of national agriculture and food policies in collaboration with the WHO Regional Office for Europe. As this was a new application of HIA, it was conducted as a pilot project (Lock, 2002; Lock et al., 2004b).

There were two aspects to this project: (i) the HIA of agriculture and nutrition policies at national level due to EU accession and the adoption of CAP; (ii) specific impacts in the rural north-east region due to the region's characteristics. Based on the results of the assessments, the HIA influenced decisions as the food security pillar was incorporated into the national FNAP.

The original policy for the HIA of food, agriculture and nutrition in Slovenia absorbed two major changes. First, the research was broadened: the original HIA covered a rural region in the north-east but this was extended to the national policy level. Although HIA priorities were re-evaluated nationally, they were designed for the characteristics of the north-east region. Second, Slovenia's negotiating positions changed many times during the process of accession to the EU (the proposed nature of EU agricultural subsidies changed regularly). Even though HIA was planned as a project to influence future national policy development, the political time frames created pressure and the provision of such support often was not possible (Lock et al., 2004a).

A five-phase HIA methodology was used: description and analysis of CAP policies and instruments; rapid appraisal workshops with stakeholders from a range of backgrounds; review of research evidence on health impacts; analysis of Slovenian data for key health-related indicators; and formation of policy recommendations for the Slovenian Government.

The methodologies employed were quantitative and qualitative. Partial economic models enabled the development of optimistic and pessimistic scenarios for the country after integrating CAP requirements (Kuhar & Erjavec, 2002); deterministic analyses of collected statistical data were applied (Lock et al., 2004b); reading materials were reviewed and workshops were held (Wallace, 2002; Lock, 2002; Gabrijelčič Blenkuš & Lock, 2004).

The first and most difficult task was to clarify which CAP policies and instruments should be considered, and what effect they would have when implemented nationally. This was not uncertain, partly because there were ongoing negotiations with the EU about the amount of CAP subsidies that Slovenia would be allocated on accession. To simplify the HIA pilot process, it was proposed to focus on a few agricultural regime spheres, as described in the text bellow, which were analysed in greater detail due to their importance in agriculture and their potentially significant health impacts (Lock et al., 2004b).

The HIA approach in Slovenia involved national and regional stakeholders. It was both multisectoral and multilevel including representatives of local farmers, food industries, consumer organizations, schools, public health organizations, nongovernmental organizations (NGOs), national and regional development agencies and officials from several government ministries (health, agriculture, finance, transport, environment, education, social affairs, work, tourism and culture) (Lock et al., 2003).

Following the HIA, several policy recommendations were made to improve health and well-being. These can be summarized in four main policy areas: fruit and vegetables, wine, dairy produce and rural development. With appropriate programmes and intersectoral collaboration, agricultural policy can be aligned with recommendations to support improvements in public health, without deviating from the primary agricultural goals. Some actions would require central changes to the CAP and are not necessarily actions that can be undertaken by the Government of Slovenia alone (Lock et al., 2004b).

The Slovenian FNAP includes the majority of the HIA's recommendations for fruit and vegetables, dairy produce and rural development. These recommendations also enabled the inclusion of the food security pillar (sustainable local food supply of health-beneficial food).

The steering group that included international experts reported to the decision-makers. Two meetings were held: one in the capital – Ljubljana; the other in the Pomurje region. The public was informed through press conferences. The project report was also discussed at the the Ministry of Agriculture, Forestry and Food, on a high political level, and presented in the Parliament.

The MoH completed the final HIA report in October 2003. It was presented to the Parliamentary Inter-Government Committee on Health in November 2003 (Lock & Gabrijelčič Blenkuš, 2004; Gabrijelčič, Zakotnik & Lock, 2004; Ministry of Health of the Republic of Slovenia, 2005). The Slovenian Parliament adopted the FNAP for Slovenia 2005–2010 unanimously in March 2005 (Ministry of Health of the Republic of Slovenia, 2005).

Aims of the HIA

From individual interviews with key informants (public health expert; civil servant in the health sector; agriculture expert; regional practitioner; regional activities coordinator) we can conclude that respondents understood the goals of the HIA. Their understanding of the aims of the HIA is based on their particular standpoints, workplace culture and level of academic education. These differing perspectives and viewpoints reveal that creating a common scientific language among various trades and overcoming semantic communication gaps take a certain amount of time. This was substantiated in the opinions of our five respondents.

The public health expert felt that, "First we wanted to see how to apply HIA to something as complex as CAP at the national level is; it was a pilot project." In the civil servant's opinion, "we wanted to influence the policy makers working with CAP, as CAP-anticipated measures could negatively reflect on the health of people." From the perspective of the agricultural expert, the aim was "quite broad, very ambitious and, because of that, unrealistic. It was well intended, but positively naive. In fact, the aim was to support Slovenian public health policy and to some extent also a broader governmental policy". The regional practitioner saw the Slovenian HIA's aim in a different way: "the intention was to harmonize agricultural and public health policies, by animating and including key partners from various ranges of other sectors". She even stated, "This was a golden opportunity for our region".

Dimensions of effectiveness

For the health, equity and community aspects, the general opinion of all the respondents was that the HIA had influenced the decision regarding FNAP, but not CAP, and raised awareness of the health aspect among decision-makers. In the words of the agricultural expert: "Perhaps the HIA, even though it did not influence the decisions, did raise the awareness of those accepting them."

Health effectiveness

The civil servant from the health sector is certain that the HIA produced changes in decision-making but cautioned that the health effects should be monitored in the long-term. The current food policy is in effect until 2010 and only then will its results be known.

The pending decision was modified and health-related changes were included with the following impacts. The food supply pillar was included uniformly in the FNAP 2005–2010 and health was considered in establishing partnerships with other sectors at regional and local levels. This project helped to ease the inclusion of health in regional developmental plans. It formed the basis of the preparation of the Mura regional developmental programme with the main aim to identify, develop and implement best practices in the field of socioeconomic and environmental development for improving the health and quality of life through different sector policies; it also enabled the implementation of the project Let's Live Healthy (health promotion in the rural area) (Buzeti, Buzeti & Belović, 2004).

The HIA raised awareness among policy-makers, although it did not affect the decision concerning CAP. It helped to develop new communication links between the ministries responsible for food, nutrition and health issues. An important side-effect was the development of the ability to understand the positions and arguments of both sides, and identify common interests. Following their discussions on the HIA, the health and agricultural sectors agreed on some common policy areas to support and implement in Slovenia after accession, for example, the future interest in rural development policy. One of the next steps was national-level intersectoral consultation involving different sectors, such as academics, NGOs and the private sector (Gregoric & Fajdiga Turk, 2005).

Equity effectiveness

The HIA focused on various vulnerable populations, monitoring and listening to certain sectors and groups, but equity was not one of the key issues of the assessment at the national level. Issues of equity were addressed more at regional level, as reflected in this interviewee's comments: "The equity issue has raised common awareness. Later on we launched projects intended to reduce health inequity. HIA had a snowball effect on understanding and perception."

We could establish that the equity aspect of the pending decision was modified mostly on the regional level. This suggests that policy-makers' awareness of equity issues was raised (for example, the Mura and Let's Live Healthy projects were granted funding).

Community effectiveness

The community aspect was also not a specific focus of the HIA, especially at national level. The regional practitioner and regional activities coordinator explained, "The community was properly informed about health consequences. The decision (inclusion of health issues in regional development plans) was changed because of our dialogue and the co-decision process." The agricultural expert and civil servant agreed that the interests of the community were taken into consideration.

The HIA project's goal was mainly to influence health but the discussions show an effect on equity and community, especially on the regional and local levels.

Discussion

Although a formal evaluation has not yet been undertaken, several important learning points have arisen from assessment of the HIA process.

Limitations of the HIA process

The two biggest problems encountered during the HIA were (i) the complexity of the agricultural policies being assessed, and (ii) the lack of robust, available evidence of the links between policy and economic and environmental conditions on one hand, and specific health impacts on the other. This required new reviews of research evidence relevant to the agricultural policy interventions being assessed. Unfortunately these were not completed as planned due to unforeseen financial and time pressures (Lock et al., 2004b).

As with many HIAs at project or policy level, this HIA was limited by pressures of time, human and financial resources. A project working group was formed at the start of this project but the lack of representatives from other sectors, particularly the Ministry of Agriculture, became a constraint for deciding policies and ensuring the involvement of stakeholders at critical points. Agricultural economists were called in to assist by joining the group.

The public health expert opinion was that broader socioeconomic determinants of health were included or were the basis for HIA. The agricultural expert opinion was that assessment was based on a relatively narrow medical concept. We conclude that there was a lack of multidisciplinary competence and that more cooperation and discussion is needed. The agricultural expert best expressed this controversy:

> … Thus one should be well versed and technically competent when dealing with intersectoral communication. Expert multidisciplinary competency is the key and we do not have enough of it. The fixation on medicine is very disturbing. Medical experts think that everything derives from it … This disrupts normal work. The agricultural experts believe that they are untouchable because of the large portion of the budget and the money they possess.

Initially the project failed to recognize the importance of ensuring familiarity with the methods or aims of HIA in Slovenia. As part of the project, a two-day HIA training course was developed but it would have been preferable to conduct the training before the start (Lock et al., 2004b).

Some Slovenian legislation covers HIA procedures, but this incorporates health only indirectly within the framework of environmental assessment and does not require an obligatory HIA. It is not required as an obligatory expert basis for political decisions therefore health issues are often overlooked in the decision-making process. We also noticed that if the HIA is not embedded in the organizational structure of decision-making bodies, benefits to intersectoral work may be reduced due to changes in the policy cycle.

Potential benefits of the HIA process

The HIA helped to develop new links between sectors, resulting in better understanding of the positions and arguments of others and identifying common interests. For all three pillars (food security, food safety and nutrition), education and raising awareness were identified as the highest priorities for the FNAP. The process would not have succeeded without the cooperation of the academics from both health and agricultural sectors. Their good relationships and substantial commitments to time and energy-consuming processes helped the work to progress.

The driving force behind the HIA came from the political level (MoH), performed by the expert level and supported by WHO. The personal involvement of the Secretary of State for Health was an important contribution to the execution of the HIA (Lock et al., 2004b). WHO Regional Office for Europe provided key support, submitting ideas and the encouragement to initiate the process.

One of the most important factors in facilitating the HIA was the change in public health culture. An interviewee confirmed this assumption:

> The culture is created through a long-term process. We managed to place health in other policies and competencies. This is an extremely vast movement. Our politicians are still not aware how big it was. It was an extraordinary event raising health to a high political level.

Key stakeholders from various non-health backgrounds also facilitated the HIA. Stakeholder workshops were considered an important mechanism for involving new participants in the decision-making process: consumers, farmers and different ministries and agencies. At local and regional levels commitments resulting from the HIA were as important as the HIA process itself. Media involvement in disseminating project results to the general public was also important.

Conclusion

In many ways, HIA of national policies is a complex process. We identified some specific factors which could contribute to the facilitation of HIA and some which could hinder the HIA process. As has been shown, HIA can not only give suggestions to help reduce potential negative and increase potential positive health influences, but also influence other aspects of the accession process.

The major benefits of the Slovenian HIA seem to be the strengthening of policy-makers' understanding of the interactions between health and other policy areas – in this case, health and agriculture – and the creation of new opportunities for improving intersectoral relationships, cooperation and understanding. The involvement of a wide range of stakeholders from different sectors broadens the issues and enables them to be considered from different viewpoints.

REFERENCES

Albreht T, et al., eds (2002). *Health care systems in transition: Slovenia.* Copenhagen, European Observatory on Health Care Systems.

Buzeti ZV, Buzeti T, Belović T (2004). *Za zdravje v deželi ob Muri. [For the health in the land down the Mura side].* Murska Sobota, Regional Institute of Public Health.

European Centre for Health Policy (1999). *Health impact assessment: main concepts and suggested approach. Gothenburg consensus paper.* Brussels, WHO Regional Office for Europe (http://www.euro.who.int/document/PAE/Gothenburgpaper.pdf, accessed 15 June 2006).

Gabrijelčič M, Zakotnik J, Lock K (2004). Health impact assessment: implementing the CAP in Slovenia after Accession. *Eurohealth*, 10(1):17–20.

Gabrijelčič Blenkuš M, Lock K (2004). Health impact assessment: historical overview and basic methodology. *Zdravstveno varstvo [Slovenian Journal of Public Health]*, 1:83–87.

Gregorič M, Fajdiga Turk V, eds (2005). *Svetovni dan hrane 2005: Lokalno trajnostna oskrba z zivili [World Food Day 2005: sustainable food supply].* Ljubljana, Institute of Public Health of the Republic of Slovenia.

Kuhar A, Erjavec E (2002). *Situation in Slovenian agricultural and food sectors and related policies with estimation of the likely future developments.* Ljubljana, Biotechnical Faculty, University of Ljubljana.

Lock K (2002). *Report of the 2nd meeting on HIA of food, agriculture and nutrition policies in Slovenia.* Rome, European Centre for Environment and Health.

Lock K (2004). Why should public health be part of an integrated European agriculture and food policy? *Eurohealth*, 10(1):1–3.

Lock K, et al. (2003) Health impact assessment (HIA) of agriculture and food policies: lessons learnt from HIA development in the Republic of Slovenia. *Bulletin of the World Health Organization*, 6:391–397.

Lock K, Gabrijelčič Blenkuš M (2004). HIA of agricultural and food policies. In: Kemm J, Parry J, Palmer S, eds. *Health impact assessment: concepts, theory, techniques and applications.* Oxford, Oxford University Press:375–387.

Lock K, et al. (2004a). Conducting health impact assessment of the effect of accession to the European Union on national agriculture and food policy in Slovenia. *Environmental Impact Assessment Review*, 24:177–188.

Lock K, et al., eds (2004b). *Health impact assessment of food and agricultural policies in Slovenia, and the potential effect of accession to the European Union: report for the Ministry of Health of the Republic of Slovenia.* Ljubljana, Ministry of Health of the Republic of Slovenia.

Ministry of Health of the Republic of Slovenia (2005). *Food and Nutrition Action Plan (FNAP) for Slovenia 2005–2010.* Ljubljana, Ministry of Health of the Republic of Slovenia.

Šelb J, Kravajna M (2000). Analiza umrljivosti v Sloveniji v letih 1987 do 1996 [Mortality rate analysis for Slovenia from 1987 to 1996]. *Zdravstveno varstvo [Slovenian Journal of Public Health]*, 39 (Suppl.):5–18.

Wallace P (2002). *HIA on food, nutrition and agriculture in Slovenia. Report of the first meeting.* Rome, European Centre for Environment and Health.

WHO Regional Office for Europe (2001). *The first action plan for food and nutrition policy 2000–2005.* Copenhagen, WHO Regional Office for Europe.

Case study 7

A private sector HIA initiative: a smoke-free workplace policy in Spain

Francisco Barroso [7]

Introduction

Until the beginning of this decade at European Union (EU) level there were few practical attempts to protect workers from environmental tobacco smoke (ETS) in workplaces (European Commission, 2004). Since then EU institutions have boosted the development of measures to prevent smoking and improve tobacco control. The European Commission was invited to propose a Council recommendation aimed at protection against involuntary exposure to tobacco smoke in public and workplaces (Council of the European Union, 2000). The Council recommended that Member States implement legislation and/or other effective measures that provide protection from exposure to ETS in indoor workplaces (Council of the European Union, 2003).

In 2001, after learning of the contents of the Conclusions of the European Council, staff in the marketing department at Mutual Cyclops (MC), a mutual insurance company,[8] decided to develop a new company service: the implementation of a workplace smoking restriction policy.

MC's executive management decided to adopt the new service within its own organization to test its performance and adapt its own working environment to the oncoming legal framework. The convenience of implementing MC's workplace smoking restriction policy and its key elements were the pending decisions of the proposal. As the new policy was going to be piloted from the

---

[7] English version reviewed by Rosa Ferrera.

[8] Mutual Cyclops is an occupational health and accident mutual insurance company which deals with more than 115 000 associated companies serving nearly 700 000 workers in Spain.

start, MC asked the Agency of Public Health of Barcelona (APHB)[9] to provide consulting services on the formulation and implementation of the policies.

The impact of the implementation of a smoke-free workplace policy was assessed between October 2001 and February 2003 (Artazcoz, Brotons & Brotons, 2003). An assessment of its health consequences was undertaken as part of the implementation test. The whole process was similar in concept and methodology to a HIA.

This case study deals with a prospective policy appraisal to assess the impact of a smoke-free workplace policy in MC, focusing on its effectiveness and the factors related to the context, inputs and processes that shaped this. This assessment was the only non-experimental prospective case found in Spain that is as recent and well documented as required for the purposes of our study.

The MC case study reveals that an HIA can be conducted with a high degree of effectiveness even without legal support, social pressure and political advocacy. Among the three dimensions considered in our research design (Blau & Wismar, 2006), the highest degree of effectiveness (direct effectiveness) was found in the community dimension. General effectiveness was found in the remaining two dimensions: equity and health.

The external context played an essential role as it provided the driving force that triggered the HIA general process. The use of applied decision aid methodology [10] (United States Department of Health and Human Services, 1997) improved the later inputs and reinforced the firm support that MC's management afforded to the whole HIA process. The company provided leadership and direction, funding and organizational means; and established new decision-making structures and processes for the assessment.

Carefully scheduled and prepared activities and the decision-maker's direct participation in the HIA process contributed to unite the assessment, decision-making process, and community involvement and dynamics. Other contextual factors improved the practice achievements.

The following section describes the impact of a smoke-free workplace policy in MC and its main characteristics.

Profile of the HIA

There is no tradition of HIA use in Spain: barely one tenth of HIA cases fitting the Gothenburg consensus (European Centre for Health Policy, 1999)

[9] The APHB is a public autonomous organization of the Sanitary Consortium of Barcelona, a consortium that coordinates and manages health centres in the capital.

[10] A guide that provides the worksite decision-makers with information on how to design, implement and evaluate ETS policies and related activities.

has been reported. There is no specific legal body for HIA in Spanish legislation; it has some consideration in the Environmental Impact Assessment Laws (JCR, 2001) but this has no effect on the practice of HIA. Political or institutional advocacy is reduced to a few manifestos at national or regional level, but no specific structural, organizational, budget or human resource support for conducting HIA has been set up widely. Only the Basque Country Regional Government actually supports an HIA experimental development initiative (Rueda, 2005). Societal support for HIA is confined to the expression of limited demands from some ecological organizations and professional associations advocating the use of HIA either individually or integrated in environmental impact assessment (EIA).

Five out of nine reported HIAs in Spain (Alonso et al., 2005) were primary research projects where no policy decisions depended on the final conclusions. The most frequent topics are those tackled most frequently by deep impact comprehensive Spanish epidemiological works and constitute a further stage of the natural development course of the technical capacities achieved within these works. They are attempts to extend these capacities to another practical field: policy decision-making.

The internal context of MC was governed by a general health concern and a deep-rooted culture of employee involvement.

Smoking in the workplace

Tobacco smoking is considered an important lifestyle determinant for individual smokers and, through passive smoking, non-smokers.

There are many policies regarding smoking in the workplace: total bans; segregated sites for smokers and non-smokers; smoke-free, with or without permit to smoke in designated outdoor locations; smoking in separately ventilated areas; smoking in designated indoor areas; outdoor-only smoking; or minor measures. MC's management decided to implement a smoke-free policy with the aim of changing the working environment and individual life-styles of 1500 employees at its 100 service centres nationwide.

The APHB were consultants for the formulation and execution of workplace smoking-restriction policies to define, assess and, subsequently, execute a proposal. The assessors proposed a smoking-cessation programme that included an assessment of its impact and the direct involvement of MC's staff.

A formal assessment steering group was set up with the main function of developing smoking policy in the workplace. Its purpose and membership were communicated to employees and managers. It comprised: MC's Director of human resources in the role of decision-maker and chairman; six employees belonging to the health and labour committees and main labour unions within the company; a middle manager charged with corporative communication and new product development; the facilities and operations manager; the company doctor; and two assessors on public health from the APHB as representatives from the public administration.

The top manager, middle manager, both APHB assessors, one employee from the health committee and an employee who did not belong to the work group were interviewed for this case study.

The impact of the implementation of a smoke-free workplace policy in MC was assessed between October 2001 and February 2003 (Artazcoz, Brotons & Brotons, 2003). The proposal was tested by applying it to a sample population of 168 stakeholders. Decreases in tobacco consumption and ETS were the assumed beneficial health impacts. The convenience and key elements of the proposal were decided upon within the working group, taking into account the results of a survey undertaken amongst all the staff at MC headquarters in Barcelona.

The methodological frame (see the UCLA School of Public Health web page at http://www.ph.ucla.edu/hs/health-impact/models.htm for further information) for the MC case was community dialogue,[11] but no formal model of HIA (Ison, 2000) was followed. The initiative was not conceived as an HIA and was not formulated as a succession of formal HIA sequential stages.

Table CS7.1 shows the time frame of the main events of the assessment regarding the pending decision. After this assessment, a smoke-free workplace policy was gradually implemented at the provision centres of MC nationwide. The main characteristics of this case are summarized in Table CS7.2.

Aims of the HIA

The interviews revealed different perceptions of the aims of the assessment and its contribution to a better decision, in contrast with unanimous agreement on its achievements. The perceptions on the aims of the process ranged from predominantly technical (pure appraisal of health outcomes) among management representatives and technical advisers to chiefly practical (improvement of health determinants) among workers. Three out of six interviewees perceived that gathering the opinions and wishes of stakeholders was an important component of the aims of this practice.

---

[11] UCLA School of Public Health research group on HIA classifies different approaches to HIA into three categories: community dialogue, quantitative analysis and bureaucratic pragmatism. The community dialogue approach focuses on public participation in decision-making, with community members actively engaged with planners in raising concerns and developing ideas for alternatives and/or in mitigating impacts.

Table CS7.1 *Time frame of the main events of the assessment regarding the pending decision*

2001	2002	2003
– Preliminary meetings (assessment starts: screening, scoping)		
– Constitution of the work group (community dynamics starts)		
– First survey (appraisal starts)		
– Initial reinforcement actions (active enforcement starts)		
– Approval of the smoke-free workplace normative (decision-making, community active dynamics ends)		
– Tested policy action starts		
– Second survey (appraisal ends, community dynamics ends)		
– Final report (assessment ends)		
		– Multicentre smoke-free policy starts

Source: Authors' compilation, based on information from interviewees.

Most of the interviewees (five out of six) granted that the method contributed to a better decision with the increased involvement of the policy-receivers; three agreed that the assessment influenced the pending decision by eliminating employees' potential attitudes of disagreement or rebuttals. This reflects the relationship between success, ownership and involvement described by Mindell and colleagues (Mindell, Ison & Joffe, 2003).

All the interviewees agreed that the MC assessment achieved its aims despite different perceptions of what these were. They observed no inconsistency between what was expected and the perceived achievements. The initiative achieved its aims and positively influenced the decision.

Dimensions of effectiveness

Health effectiveness

As five out of six interviewees stated, the MC assessment was commonly considered to achieve general health effectiveness. All the interviewees acknowledged adequate consideration of health in the decision-making process, but only two accepted that the pending decision was modified according to health aspects. Most of the interviewees (four out of six), stated that there

Table CS7.2 *Main characteristics of the case on the impact of a smoke-free workplace policy in Mutual Cyclops*

Year of completion:	2003 (Time of assessment: October 2001–February 2003)
National context for HIA	
Use of HIA:	No tradition of HIA use. Few experimental HIA cases conducted, very few real HIA conducted.
Technical capacity:	Appraisal capacity well developed but few or no human resources trained to conduct specific HIA.
General characteristics	
Type:	Comprehensive, prospective HIA.
Sector:	Services
Topic:	Lifestyle, workplace indoor pollution
Geographical location:	Assessment: sub-local, urban area, workplace. Decision: multicentre at national level, urban, workplaces.
Characteristics of the decision	
Pending decision:	Implementing a workplace smoking cessation policy and its key elements.
Policy options:	Theoretical: from no action or minor measures to total bans. Practical: no action versus smoke-free policy versus separately ventilated areas.
Policy formulation:	Adjustment to existing possibilities: consulting and negotiating with interested parties.
Decision magnitude:	Modifying workplace conditions and workers' habits in a service company workplace (policy receivers: 1500 employees of Mutual Cyclops nationwide).
Methodology-related characteristics	
Assessment health indicators:	ETS occupational exposure, tobacco consumption prevalence and number of cigarettes smoked per day.
Risk assessment:	No
Evidence used as input:	Comparison with the results of available policy options, obtained from systematic reviews of scientific literature.

Source: Author's compilation.

was no need for the pending decision to be modified as the definition of the policy was based on the results of the assessment process. Those with a technical perception of the assessment felt that the health outcomes obtained were better than expected and very satisfactory. The initiative was considered to be an effective means to define a health policy.

Equity effectiveness

The method was commonly considered to have achieved general equity effectiveness (five out of six interviewees). Again, all the interviewees endorsed adequate acknowledgement of equity in the decision-making process, although two stated that this was not explicit. According to these actors, the equity of the policy was assured by the heterogeneity of stakeholders in the working group that defined the key elements of the policy; the possibility that policy-receivers could participate directly in the decision-making (by means of the survey); and the equitable distribution of restrictions and enforcement across all job categories.

Harris-Roxas and colleagues considered community participation and application of principles emphasizing equity, i.e. equity and social justice, to be explicit mechanisms for incorporating equity in HIA (Harris-Roxas, Simpson & Harris, 2004). For these interviewees equity was never a necessity to develop the assessment, but a characteristic of the company's culture and an implicit concept that configures the applied method (United States Department of Health and Human Services, 1997). Five interviewees certified that the pending decision did not have to be modified for equity as this was intrinsic in the decision-making process through the principles of equity and social justice or community participation. The initiative was considered to be an effective instrument in incorporating equity into the policy.

Community effectiveness

By consensus, the MC assessment was considered to attain direct community effectiveness: the community's interests were acknowledged adequately in the decision-making process. The pending decision was modified, or even defined, by taking account of the opinions, interest, preferences or wishes of the employees.

The MC managers considered direct participation of the policy-receivers in the decision-making process to be a prerequisite for implementing the smoke-free policy (even granting them power to veto the initiative). The employees were consulted by means of an individual survey, and the choice of the majority concerning the type of ETS policy was incorporated in the decisions of the working group. Decisions made within the working group are attributable to the assessment – an instrument of policy-resolution and definition. Policy-receivers' interests accounted for an early and critical stage of policy formulation and the assessment achieved a high degree of community effectiveness.

Process, context and input of HIA

Process

Although not conceived as an HIA, the initiative was designed to integrate with the policy-making process as Kemm considered HIA should do (Kemm,

2001). The scheme of the process was outlined in advance [12] and presented as a proposal at the meeting to form the working group; therefore its members ratified the proposal.

The tight-focus foregoing approach for this evidence-based policy assessment contrasts with the community dialogue methodological framework referred to in the assessment-profiling section. In fact, this approach was not exclusive. Informal knowledge from opinion surveys [13] was also used as evidence for the assessment in the policy definition stage, modulating the reliance on the tight-focus foregoing approach towards a more broad-focused approach (Kemm, 2001). This observes the principle of openness (Kemm, 2003) and community involvement in the decision-making process enhances its legitimacy. As Kemm has argued (Kemm, 2003), the assessment acts as a factor that supplies general effectiveness by increasing the decision-makers' sense of ownership.

The appraisal was conceived as a formal stage. Occupational environment and lifestyle were considered, by consensus, as health determinants to be affected by the decision,[14] but there was no explicit and concrete initial evaluation of the expected health gain in terms of ETS exposure or decreased tobacco consumption. The interviewees were in general agreement about the initial consensus on the expected benefits and the lack of expected negative outcomes. This agreement extended to their judgments about policy-receivers' positive perception on the effects of pending decisions. This reflects the assessment's public health advocacy effect, its influence on public opinion and capacity to shape policy-maker's judgements, as Kemm pointed out (Kemm, 2001). The health advocacy capacity of the assessment is recognized here as a factor that improves health effectiveness.

The evidence for the appraisal was obtained by comparing the health outcomes of the assessed policy implementation with those from similar initiatives, by systematic review of scientific literature. Mindell et al. discussed the type and quality of evidence used in HIA (Mindell et al., 2004). The APHB coordinator communicated results in a presentation to the executive company manager of MC in the course of a formal meeting; general information was relayed through a campaign coordinated by the middle manager. This resulted in the

---

[12] Scoping and screening procedures took place at some preliminary meetings between MC management and APHB representatives before the working group was set up. Only potential beneficial impacts were outlined and identified applying the criteria of certainty of impact and measurability of impacts. The selection criterion for the target population was geographical proximity. Targeted groups were defined by means of smoking status, age and gender criteria. The functional approach and scope of the assessment, including the methodology, and the spatial and temporal scales defining the impact were proposed at these meetings.

[13] These surveys consisted of anonymous questionnaires to each member of staff; Artazcoz et al. described them and their results (Artazcoz, Brotons & Brotons et al., 2003).

[14] Passive exposure to ETS, smoking prevalence and tobacco consumption among smokers were the health indicators used for the appraisal. MC assessment design was a longitudinal pre-test/post-test; two repeated measures on a single sample group design, constituting this design a quasi-experiment.

dissemination of the survey results to every employee. These methods fulfilled the formal and functional needs of the decision-makers and, by meeting their requirements, improved the capacity to influence them.

All the interviewees understood that employee empowerment in the decision-making process was the main factor for improving community effectiveness. Three interviewees remarked that the surveys helped to increase credibility for the policy-receivers. Four interviewees agreed that keeping employees informed throughout the entire process[15] produced the same effect. However, none of them recognized transparency or credibility as factors that improved community effectiveness.

Davenport and colleagues (Davenport, Mathers & Parry, 2006) identified balance between decision-maker ownership and HIA credibility to be an enabler for integrating HIA findings into decision-making. The incorporation of informal knowledge by means of participative events and information dynamics increased policy-receivers' perception of ownership and credibility of the process and enhanced community effectiveness.

Community dynamics started at an early stage of the assessment with formal ratification of the intervention strategy by employees' representatives within the working group. WHO has emphasized the importance of early involvement (European Centre for Health Policy, 1999).

A sequence of indirect (contribution of employees' representatives within the working group) and direct participative interventions (two direct consultations conducted before and after the execution of the assessed policy) were made. The community received feedback at every stage of its intervention by way of a series of passive (information) and active (smoking-cessation therapies) reinforcement measures and smoking restrictions. Sorensen and colleagues remarked on the importance of reinforcement on worksite smoking-cessation policies (Sorensen, Lando & Pechacek, 1993).

There was a consensus among interviewees on the nature and convenience of the applied reinforcement measures and their equity.[16] However, although restrictions were applied equally across job categories, only one interviewee noted the effect on perceived equity. Equitable distribution of reinforcements and restrictions appear as the main equity-effectiveness factors.

The sequence of community participative events and its feedback transformed the initiative into a very interactive process for the community. Among the

[15] The communication of the information on health-related decisions taken within the working group was coordinated and channelled by MC's doctor.

[16] The main reinforcement measures applied were a continuous information campaign, controlled access to smoking-cessation therapy groups, individual hotline therapy support, and reimbursement of substitutive therapy costs in cases of successful smoking cessation.

stakeholders it produced a long-term interest in the general process as indicated by the high response rate to the second survey. In the case of MC, the interactivity constitutes an important instrumental enabler for community effectiveness.

Community dynamics directly influenced the decision-making process. Decision-making resulted in a sequential transfer of information and decision-making authority up, down and up again through the MC hierarchy. The executive company manager made the decision to test the new service proposal. The convenience of the initiative model proposed by the APHB coordinator was decided by the HR manager and ratified by community representatives. The community decided on the convenience of the assessed policy and the HR manager ratified its definition. The executive company manager ratified the decision based on its convenience for implementing the assessed policy nationwide.

Democracy value (European Centre for Health Policy, 1999) expressed here by a decision made jointly increased the acceptability of the final decision. Community dynamics acts here as a health and community effectiveness factor as suggested by Kauppinen and colleagues (Kauppinen, Nelimarkka & Pertillä, 2006).

Context

In the absence of national, regional or local governance to stimulate the assessment, the confluence of external and internal contextual circumstances discussed in the assessment-profiling section acted as a trigger input. However, interviewees reported differing opinions on the nature of the issues that activated the initiative: from the lack of explicit intention to conduct an HIA to the need to adapt the organization before an oncoming legal framework. In the case of MC, a health intervention assessment or a new company service test was transformed into an HIA matching the Gothenburg consensus by the use of applied decision-aid methodology (United States Department of Health and Human Services, 1997) proposed by APHB assessors.

The methodology applied in MC provided a structured framework to develop leadership, commitment, direction and organizational means as basic inputs for a proper assessment and policy implementation. These included obtaining management commitment and support; offering support to employees; providing middle managers and supervisors with training in policy communication and enforcements; providing real and visible opportunities for employee participation in policy-planning and implementation; facilitating access to the policy formulation to formal or informal working groups; and ensuring that restrictions and enforcement were equitable across job categories. It also focused these practices on stakeholders' involvement and equity for policy-receivers.

Other guidelines, such as establishing formal or informal working groups with representatives of employees and the decision-maker, taking account of employees' opinions, and thoughtful planning and sequential introduction of the policy also contributed to integrate the decision-making process with impact assessment and community dynamics as key structuring inputs. Some of these guidelines are related to community effectiveness. There is remarkable coincidence among the values that govern this method, HIA and the internal context of MC. Davenport and colleagues cited the use of a consistent methodological approach as a technical enabler for integrating HIA findings into the decision-making process (Davenport, Mathers & Parry, 2006).

Input

Davenport and colleagues also cited congruency between HIA timing and the decision-making process as another technical enabler for successful integration of HIA findings (Davenport, Mathers & Parry, 2006). This technical input and design of detailed planning that incorporated the three practices (decision-making, impact assessment and community dynamics) were confirmed by the managers and technical assessors consulted. Workers representatives agreed with these statements and believed that impact-assessment results – including recommendations and the opinions and preferences of stakeholders – were communicated correctly to the decision-makers. However, they found it more difficult to give more details about the decision-making process. All the interviewees acknowledged that stakeholders' participation was made possible by early involvement.

The enabling effect of technical input seems to be clear. Moreover, the capability of the MC organization to internalize APBH consultancy rises as a functional input that contributes to the general effectiveness.

Nevertheless, it is difficult to profile the relevance of other inputs to the assessment. Interviewees disagreed about the significance or differential weight of the role that any person played as a leading or driving force in the initiative. Only management representatives and technical advisers recognized their individual tasks to be membership of working groups. None of the interviewed workers considered that they had assumed an individual role. Management staff identified the community or its representatives as the origins of driving force or sources for directions and leadership; workers not only stressed that the origins were with the company managers, but also denied any leadership from the community. Technical advice, moderating, linking and coordination roles were acknowledged by APHB staff and MC's managers. Most of the interviewed actors (four out of six) recognized that company managers were the origin of the commitment. All of them alluded to the support from MC top management, giving its initial consent, assisting the whole process or assuming the costs.

The transfer of decision-making authority across the hierarchy of the company and the multiplicity of specific tasks of the memberships within the working group may explain the lack of perceived relevance of driving forces, leadership and directions. With proper commitment, an organization like MC may substitute the driving forces and leadership needed for the assessment with its intrinsic organizational and functional capacity.

The formal constitution and operation of the working group represent a relevant organizational and functional input linked to community effectiveness. Decisions were entailed in the context of the formulation and implementation of a workplace smoking policy. The group was formed to initiate a participation process that promoted consensus and avoided eventual conflicts when implementing a certain non-smoking normative. No interviewee referred to any opinion against the process or controversy over it.

Conclusion

The MC assessment was a means to bring health into all the determinants and improve the health impacts of the smoke-free workplace policy implemented in this company. It progressed in the absence of statutory mandates for HIA and constitutes a case of a voluntary HIA developed in a mutual insurance company.

Stakeholders considered that the assessment achieved high effectiveness. The resolution to define and implement a smoke-free workplace policy is attributable to the assessment. The HIA improved decision-makers' legitimacy and ownership; increased policy-receivers' credibility and ownership; influenced decision-makers and policy-receivers; and exercised health advocacy for both. The internal context of MC acted as a triggering factor of the assessment and enabled the application of a structuring method consistent with HIA values.

Small to medium workplaces where occupational health initiatives are executed regularly may offer appropriate situations for the exercise of effective HIA.

REFERENCES

Alonso E, et al. (2005). Health impact evaluation of particle air pollution in five Spanish cities: European APHEIS Project. *Revista Española de Salud Pública*, 79(2):297–308.

Artazcoz L, Brotons M, Brotons A (2003). Impacto de la implantación de una política de trabajo libre de humo en una empresa. *Gaceta Sanitaria*, 17(6):490–493.

Blau J, Wismar M (2006). Conceptual framework and key results from the effectiveness of health impact assessment project. *European Journal of Public Health*, 16(Suppl.1):86.

The Council of the European Union (2000). Council conclusions of 18 November 1999 on combating tobacco consumption (2000/C 86/03). *Official Journal of the European Communities*, 24 March:C86/4-C86/5.

The Council of the European Union (2003). Council recommendation of 2 December 2002 on the prevention of smoking and on initiatives to improve tobacco control (2003/54/EC). *Official Journal L022*, 25 January:0031–0034.

Davenport C, Mathers J, Parry J (2006). Use of health impact assessment in incorporating health considerations in decision-making. *Journal of Epidemiology and Community Health*, 60:196–201.

European Centre for Health Policy (1999). *Health impact assessment: main concepts and suggested approach. Gothenburg consensus paper.* Brussels, WHO Regional Office for Europe (http://www.euro.who.int/document/PAE/Gothenburgpaper.pdf, accessed 15 June 2006).

European Commission (2004). *Tobacco or health in the European Union – past, present and future.* Luxembourg, Office for Official Publications of the European Communities.

Harris-Roxas B, Simpson S, Harris E (2004). *Equity focused health impact assessment: a literature review.* Sydney, Centre for Health Equity Training Research and Evaluation (CHETRE) on behalf of the Australasian Collaboration for Health Equity Impact Assessment (ACHEIA).

Ison E (2000). *A resource for health impact assessment: Volume 1 (the main resource). Part III: Resources for health impact assessment. Section 6: Models of HIA.* London, Commissioned by the NHS Executive (http://www.londonshealth.gov.uk/pdf/r_hia6.pdf, accessed 05 June 2006).

JCR (2001). *LEY 6/2001, de 8 de mayo, de modificación del Real Decreto legislativo 1302/1986, de 28 de junio, de evaluación de impacto ambiental [ACT 6/2001, of May, the 8th, on modifying the Royal Legislative Act 1302/1986, on June the 28th, on Environment Impact Assessment].* BOE n.111 09/05/2001:16607–16616.

Kauppinen T, Nelimarkka K, Pertillä K (2006). A case-study of the role of health impact assessment in implementing welfare strategy at local level. In: Ståhl T, et al., eds. *Health in all policies: prospects and potentials.* Helsinki, Finnish Ministry of Social Affairs and Health:263–266.

Kemm J (2001). Health impact assessment: a tool for healthy public policy. *Health Promotion International*, 16(1):79–85.

Kemm J (2003). Perspectives on health impact assessment. *Bulletin of the World Health Organization*, 81(6):387.

Mindell J, Ison E, Joffe M (2003). A glossary for health impact assessment. *Journal of Epidemiology and Community Health*, 57:647–651.

Mindell J, et al. (2004). Enhancing the evidence base for health impact assessment. *Journal of Epidemiology and Community Health*, 58:546–551.

Rueda JR (2005). *Guía para la evaluación del impacto en la salud y en el bienestar de proyectos, programmeas o políticas extrasanitarias: Investigación Comisionada [Guidelines for assessing the impact of projects, programmes or non-health policies on health and well-being of individuals.*

Commissioned research]. Vitoria-Gasteiz. Departamento de Sanidad. Gobierno Vasco. Informe nº: Osteba D-05-04. Salud pública. I. Euskadi. Departamento de Sanidad. II. Título. III. Serie. 614.

Sorensen G, Lando H, Pechacek TF (1993). Promoting smoking cessation at the workplace. Results of a randomized controlled intervention study. *Journal of Occupational and Medicine*, 35(2):121–126.

UCLA School of Public Health (DATE). Health Impact Assessment. Information and Insight for Policy Decisions. Methodology: Models (taxonomy of HIA) [web site]. Washington, D.C., UCLA School of Public Health (http://www.ph.ucla.edu/hs/health-impact/models.htm, accessed 28 March 2007).

United States Department of Health and Human Services (1997). *Making your workplace smoke free. A decision-maker's guide*. Washington, D.C., Centers for Disease Control and Prevention, Office on Smoking and Health, Wellness Councils of America, American Cancer Society.

Case study 8

HIA speeding up the decision-making process: the reconstruction of route 73 in Sweden

Ida Knutsson and Anita Linell[17]

Introduction

The case study for Sweden focuses on a health impact assessment (HIA) performed when planning for a new Route 73 – the main trunk road between Stockholm and the port of Nynäshamn. The case study was selected for several reasons. It:

- is well documented;

- was performed recently therefore it was easy to find relevant actors and stakeholders for interviews;

- includes an interesting decision-making process. Some stakeholders protested against the construction of a new Route 73. The decision whether to construct a new route in accordance with the proposed solution therefore was made by the Swedish Ministry of Sustainable Development and ultimately the Swedish Government;

- is based on the new Swedish public health policy which includes objectives and determinants and outlines prioritized groups.

During the study, six interviewees representing different actors and stakeholders involved in the decision-making process were contacted. Their opinions are the basis for the conclusions in this case study. The analysis of effectiveness is

---

[17] Anita Linell was involved in the steering group of the HIA of Route 73.

based on a partial HIA which is part of the environmental impact assessment (EIA), and a complementary HIA performed in accordance with the new public health policy. The case study not only shows the effectiveness of the partial HIA but also presents the benefits of developing it into an HIA in accordance with the new guidelines in Sweden, i.e. the new public health policy and the Guideline on HIA published by The Swedish National Institute of Public Health (SNIPH, 2005a).

Profiling the HIA

Health issues are being allocated increasingly higher priority on the decision-making agenda in Sweden. The Swedish Parliament (The Riksdag) recently adopted a bill for public health and a strategy for sustainable development (SNIPH, 2003).

- In 2003 the Riksdag adopted 11 national objectives for public health as part of a new strategy for addressing public health and social sustainability.

- The overall aim of Swedish public health policy is to create social conditions which ensure good health on equal terms for the entire population.

- It has been established that improving the public health of those groups most vulnerable to ill-health is particularly important.

- Evidence-based health determinants were chosen as the basis for the policy. The benefit of using determinants instead of health outcomes as a basis for political decisions is that ill-health can be avoided more easily.

- SNIPH has developed further the indicators for monitoring each objective.

- During the last few years, the Government has commissioned a number of central agencies to develop an HIA methodology and perform HIA within their fields. SNIPH has been instructed to support the agencies with this task.

Even if public health policy has been strengthened on the national level in the last few years, Sweden has a lot to implement before public health is considered to be of equal importance to economic and labour market policy respectively (SNIPH, 2003).

HIA in the case study – an explanation

In Sweden, an EIA contains an HIA as a legal requirement of the Environmental Code. This kind of HIA is focused on environmental health determinants; equity is very seldom assessed and the gender perspective is analysed sparsely. Health analyses are often presented in different chapters of the reports and usually not summarized. This was the case in the EIA for

Table CS8.1 *A matrix showing how different health variables of Route 73 are considered in partial HIA (EIA) and HIA*

Assessment/ Health aspects	EIA including a partial HIA	Complementary HIA in accordance with the new public health policy
Determinants/indicators	Environmental health determinants	Environmental health determinants + relevant public health (social) determinants
Equity and prioritized groups	Not systematically analysed	Systematically analysed
Gender perspective	Assessed for some of the determinants	Assessed for all relevant determinants
Presentation of health aspects	Health analyses in different chapters of the report	Summarized presentation in the report

Source: SNIPH, 2005b; Swedish Road Administration, 2002.

Route 73 and the reason why the health analysis in the EIA is called a partial HIA in this case study.

The complementary HIA which was performed in accordance with the new public health policy in Sweden includes both social and environmental health determinants, equity and gender perspective. Also, all the health aspects are presented together to give the decision-makers an overview. Table CS8.1 shows how different health aspects were assessed in the partial HIA of Route 73 and the HIA in accordance with the new public health policy.

HIA in accordance with the new public health policy is based on the Gothenburg consensus definition. According to this, the overall aim of an HIA is to provide planners and decision-makers with knowledge about the possible health effects of a political decision. This may be a decision regarding projects, plans, programmes, activities or individual draft measures. An HIA should help to provide a better basis for decision-making and be used to influence decisions in order to safeguard public health. An HIA constitutes a good tool for highlighting how new political decisions contribute to the attainment of both environmental and social sustainability (SNIPH, 2005a).

Route 73

Route 73 between Stockholm and Nynäshamn includes a 25 km stretch of road that is very dangerous (SNIPH, 2005b) and is sometimes referred to as "the road of death". The traffic load is very high in relation to the condition of the road and the flow of traffic is gradually increasing – in 2020 this is expected to have increased by about 70%. Route 73 is classified as a road of both national and regional interest because it connects the mainland with the island of Gotland and eastern Europe. It is also important for the traffic flow between Nynäshamn and Södertörn (the southern suburbs of Stockholm).

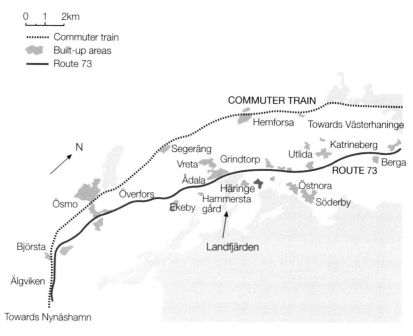

Figure CS8.1 *Map showing the zero alternative for Route 73*
Source: Swedish Road Administration, 2002.

Currently the road passes through a landscape of considerable natural and cultural value (see Figure CS8.1). There are sensitive coastal areas on one side of the road and forest and other natural environments that are important for outdoor life and recreation on the other.

Several alternative solutions to address the increasing traffic problems but protect the natural and cultural values as far as possible were considered. The EIA by the Regional Road Administration of Stockholm analysed seven different alternatives for a new stretch of road. The findings resulted in the recommendation of alternative E for the new stretch of road (see Figure CS8.2). This proposes a four-lane road including a by-pass (stretch A–B in Figure CS8.2) running through a recreation area. The existing Route 73 will be rebuilt as a local road, with room for footpaths and cycle paths and access to public transport.

The decision-making process

The decision-making process for the Route 73 construction project is described on a timeline shown in Figure CS8.3. This also shows the role of the interviewees in the study. The numbered circles represent the interviewees and their roles in the decision-making process.

In 2000, the Regional Road Administration of Stockholm initiated a construction project on Route 73. In accordance with the Environmental

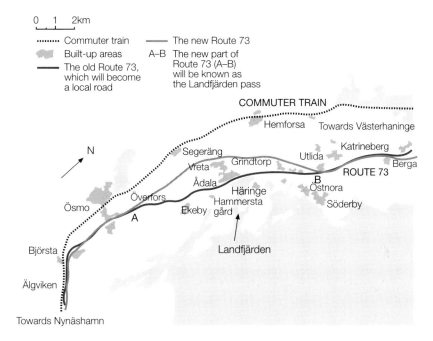

Figure CS8.2 *Map showing alternative E for the new Route 73*
Source: Swedish Road Administration, 2002.

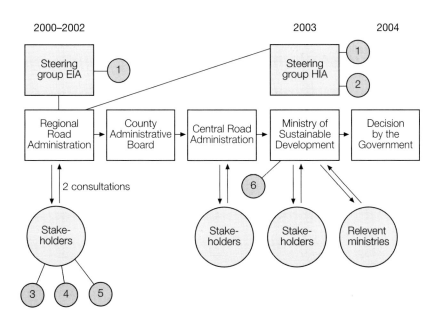

Figure CS8.3 *Schematic figure showing the decision-making process of Route 73 on a timeline*

Code, they were required to perform an EIA in order to apply for permission for the construction. The code stipulates what is expected from the EIA, including how the planned project will affect human health – partial HIA (see Table CS8.1). The Regional Road Administration instructed consultants to carry out the EIA but maintained responsibility for its quality. The County Administrative Board in each county is the final decision-maker for road traffic projects in Sweden, in this case the County of Stockholm.

The Environmental Code requires the EIA to be sent to and scrutinized by different stakeholders affected by the project (central and regional agencies, municipalities, organizations with interests in the issue and private stakeholders) before it is complete. The Regional Road Administration accomplished this by means of hearings and exhibitions during the EIA process and by sending out review copies of the EIA to the stakeholders.

The Swedish Environmental Protection Agency (SEPA) expressed concerns about the construction during the review of the EIA. The Agency felt that the project was in conflict with the national environmental quality objectives set by the Riksdag. The new stretch of road would run too close to the protected natural areas and encroach on recreational green areas. The final decision on the construction of a new stretch of Route 73 therefore had to be settled by the Ministry of Sustainable Development and, ultimately, the Swedish Government.

The decision date was postponed several times by the Ministry of Sustainable Development. When actors and stakeholders expressed concern about the lengthy wait an officer at the Municipality of Nynäshamn suggested an HIA as an effective tool to speed up the decision-making process. They contacted SNIPH and expressed an interest in cooperating on a complementary HIA for Route 73. The HIA in accordance with the new public health policy was initiated in 2003 by SNIPH, the Municipality of Nynäshamn and the Regional Road Administration of Stockholm.

This complementary HIA focused on a comparison between alternative E (Figure CS8.2) and the zero alternative (Figure CS8.1). In February 2004 the Ministry of Sustainable Development and the Government made the decision to permit the construction of Route 73 according to alternative E. The results of the complementary HIA strengthened alternative E's case as the best solution although the final report was not published until 2005.

Actors and stakeholders

The steering group of the complementary HIA comprised representatives from SNIPH, the Regional Road Administration of Stockholm and the Municipality of Nynäshamn, and met on six occasions. They led the HIA-process, conducted the analysis and put the results in writing. SNIPH was the administrative coordinator of the group. During the course of the complementary HIA, including the final report, a large reference group comprising representatives from central agencies, county councils, municipalities and research organizations submitted comments.

The interviewees in this case study pointed out different stakeholders affected by the decision-making process. The stakeholders included not only central agencies and the County Administrative Board, but also municipalities (especially the Municipality of Nynäshamn) and other local stakeholders. The list of local stakeholders included residents in the affected area, amounting to about 5000 people in 2002 (Swedish Road Administration, 2002); road-users (normal road-users including pedestrians, commuters to Stockholm and road-users for the ferries in Nynäshamn); people who enjoy outdoor recreation in the area (horse-riders, hunters etc.); local businesses, organizations and societies.

Two organizations, each represented by an interviewee, were of special interest in the case study. The local Green Party in Nynäshamn opposed the construction because they believe transport problems to be a global concern; the best solution to the problems on Route 73 would be to spend money on public transport, preferably by improving the commuter train network. Route 73 Now was a local initiative in Nynäshamn that lobbied in favour of the construction. It focused on items of local interest in the alternatives, such as improved commercial traffic and local health aspects. During the decision-making process Route 73 Now had fought to include worry and insecurity about the risk of accidents in the partial HIA, but received little recognition for this.

Guidelines for HIA in Sweden

SNIPH has been tasked by the Swedish Government to develop HIA methods in accordance with the new public health policy within a number of strategically important areas and to support the application of HIA at central, regional and local levels. The Institute has published a general guide on how to conduct an HIA (SNIPH, 2005a). This method is to be seen as an existing formal model in Sweden.

The method builds on the objectives for environmental and social (public health) sustainability and encompasses five general steps:

1 screening
2 scoping
3 appraisal
4 results and recommendations
5 monitoring and evaluation.

According to the national policy on public health in Sweden, it is not sufficient for an HIA merely to assess the extent to which the population will be affected. It is important to ensure that differences in ill-health are not increased therefore groups that suffer from, or are at risk of, poor health are studied. These are referred to as prioritized or vulnerable groups. Some issues should always be considered when examining how a decision affects health equity (Government of Sweden, 2002):

- age
- ethnicity
- socioeconomic background
- sexual orientation
- disability
- gender.

In the partial HIA of Route 73, prioritized groups were not analysed systematically (see Table CS8.1). This was one motive for conducting an HIA in accordance with the new public health policy. In the complementary HIA of Route 73, the selected priority groups were children, adults/professionals, older people, people with disabilities, chronically ill persons, horse-riders and hunters. The effects on the population as a whole were also considered.

In the assessments for the complementary HIA the health matrix was used as a basis for demonstrating how a decision affects attainment of the various objectives and how it impacts on different vulnerable groups (SNIPH, 2005b). The assessments in the HIA were performed in three different environments for both alternative E and the zero alternative: (i) traffic; (ii) living; (iii) recreational.

The determinants used to assess the environmental and social effects of the alternatives in each environment were based on the public health and environmental quality objectives adopted by the Riksdag. Examples of the assessments performed in the complementary HIA of Route 73 can be found in Figures CS8.4 and CS8.5 below (SNIPH, 2005b).

Aims of the HIA

The aim of the partial HIA in the EIA was to fulfil the mandatory regulations of the Environmental Code (see Table CS8.1).

The aims of the complementary HIA of Route 73 were to:

Objectives and determinants		Children	Adults/ profession-als	Older people	Persons with disabilities	Chroni-cally persons	Com-mercial drivers	Entire popu-lation
Priority groups →								

PUBLIC HEALTH OBJECTIVES

Objectives and determinants		Children	Adults/ professionals	Older people	Persons with disabilities	Chronically persons	Commercial drivers	Entire population
Safe environments and products	Injuries in the traffic environment (risk)	◆	◆	◆	◆		◆	
	Transportation of hazardous goods (risk)	◆		◆		◆	◆	
	Worry/insecurity about the risk of accident		◆				◆	
Increased physical activity	Supportive environments for physical activity	◆	◆	◆	◆		...	

ENVIRONMENTAL OBJECTIVES

		Children	Adults/ professionals	Older people	Persons with disabilities	Chronically persons	Commercial drivers	Entire population
Clean air	Nitrogen dioxide levels	◆		◆		◆	...	
	Particle levels	◆		◆		◆	...	
	Hydrogen levels	◆		◆		◆	...	
Good built environment	Noise	◆		◆	◆	◆	...	

Unchanged	Improvement	Deterioration/Change for the worse

··· = Not relevant   ◆ = Priority groups standing to gain/lose considerably as a result of the decision

Figure CS8.4 *Assessment of the traffic environment year 2020 for alternative E* [18]

- supplement and magnify the partial HIA performed in the Route 73 EIA.

- show how an HIA can highlight how new political decisions contribute to the attainment of social sustainability by analysing social determinants and equity.

- provide planners and decision-makers with knowledge about the possible health effects of the alternatives, both physical and mental.

- to show how HIA can be applied in a road traffic project.

Dimensions of effectiveness

The results in the effectiveness analysis focus on the partial HIA but the conclusions also reflect the benefits gained from performing an HIA in accordance with the new public health policy.

---

[18] A corresponding assessment was made for the zero alternative in order to make it easy for decision-makers to compare the alternatives. The assessment is made in relation to the present situation.

Objectives and determinants		Children	Adults/ professionals	Older people	Persons with disabilities	Chronically persons	Commercial drivers	Entire population
PUBLIC HEALTH OBJECTIVES								
Safe environments and products	Injuries in the traffic environment (risk)	...	...	...	...	...	...	...
	Transportation of hazardous goods (risk)	♦		♦		♦	...	
	Worry/insecurity about the risk of accident		♦				...	
Increased physical activity	Supportive environments for physical activity	♦	♦	♦	♦	♦	...	
ENVIRONMENTAL OBJECTIVES								
Reduced climate impact	Carbon dioxide emissions						...	
Clean air	Nitrogen dioxide levels	♦		♦		♦	...	
	Particle levels	♦		♦		♦	...	
	Hydrogen levels	♦		♦		♦	...	
Non-toxic environment	Spread of persistent organic pollutants and heavy metals	♦	♦				...	
Good-quality groundwater	Leakage of road salt/chloride	♦					...	
Good-build environment	Noise	♦		♦	♦	♦	...	
	Vibrations						...	
	Accessibility	♦		♦	♦		...	
	Encroachment on cultural environment/ green areas						...	
Flourishing lakes and streams	Scope for recreation							
Sustainable forests	Scope for recreation						♦	

Unchanged   Improvement   Deterioration/Change for the worse

... = Not relevant   ♦ = Priority groups standing to gain/lose considerably as a result of the decision

Figure CS8.5 *Assessment of the living and recreational environments, alternative E in 2020* [19]

Health effectiveness

Three interviewees considered that the partial HIA had general health effectiveness (see matrix on dimensions of effectiveness in the framework for the project "Effectiveness of Health Impact Assessment" (European

---

[19] A corresponding assessment was made for the zero alternative in order to make it easy for decision-makers to compare the alternatives. The assessment is made in relation to the present situation.

Observatory on Health Systems and Policies, 2005)). The primary reason given was that the health outcomes from the decision were positive. Health aspects, i.e. exposure to air pollution, exposure to noise and risk of accidents, were affected positively by the choice of alternative E.

The interviewee representing an adviser to the decision-makers stated that the partial HIA had general health effectiveness since it would not have been possible to reach a decision without it. This is mandatory in the Environmental Code.

One interviewee stated that the partial HIA had direct health effectiveness as some changes were made to the proposal during the process because of presumed health effects.

One benefit of the complementary HIA is that it deepened public-health awareness among practitioners, stakeholders and decision-makers by addressing not only environmental determinants but also social determinants and equity. Another benefit stated by one of the interviewees was that mental health, worry and insecurity about accidents were now included although they had experienced difficulties in getting this included in the partial HIA. The complementary HIA also included the social determinant of supportive environments for physical activity.

Equity effectiveness

Interviewees gave different answers about equity effectiveness. Three felt that it was not relevant, possibly because implementation of the new public health policy has just started and they felt that they had too little knowledge about equity to answer the question.

One interviewee said that the partial HIA had general equity effectiveness, either because equity consequences were of negligible importance in the decision or because the equity consequences from the decision were positive. Another stated that the partial HIA had no effectiveness in equity aspects because it lacked a systematic analysis of prioritized groups and the decision did not take such issues into account. One interviewee stated that the partial HIA had direct equity effectiveness because changes had been made during the hearings in the EIA process.

The complementary HIA considered and analysed prioritized groups thereby helping to raise awareness of equity amongst practitioners, stakeholders and decision-makers.

Community effectiveness

Once again interviewees had divided opinions. Two answered that the partial HIA had general community effectiveness as the community had been informed adequately about health consequences. During the decision-making process, there had been at least two public hearings and a few exhibitions about the planned project that gave the community opportunities to learn about the consequences of the alternatives.

Two interviewees stated that the partial HIA had direct community effectiveness, since the alternative solutions had been modified due to dialogue with the community. For example, the interests of horse-riders and hunters had been protected as a result of giving them the opportunity to express their concerns. Concerns raised during the hearings and exhibitions were also considered adequately by the decision-makers.

Two interviewees answered that the question was not relevant for them because they had not been involved in the consultation process.

Other dimensions of effectiveness

Other dimensions of effectiveness mentioned by the interviewees included cost, decision and administrative effectiveness respectively. The interviewees saw that these dimensions were applicable to HIA in general terms.

According to the interviewees, HIA is cost-effective because it helps to eliminate bad alternatives and leads to resources being invested in health-improving alternatives. HIA is also decision-effective since it helps to point out the best alternative and provides a thorough assessment of the possible solutions.

Administrative effectiveness refers to the effective meeting between competences in the society at large and those within central agencies. One interviewee stated that "What is not written is often just as important as what is", in other words, the process itself, whereby competences meet and experience is built up, is equally as important as the result.

Conclusion

Dimensions of effectiveness

The effectiveness analysis in this case study is focused on the partial HIA performed in the EIA of Route 73. Interviewees also commented on the benefits of performing a complementary HIA in accordance with the new public health policy.

The case study of Route 73 shows that the partial HIA had general health effectiveness and general or direct community effectiveness. For equity effectiveness, the answers were less easy to interpret as they were all different. In summary, according to the interviewees, equity was not very high on the partial HIA agenda because the decision-makers and actors lacked awareness of such issues.

If the complementary HIA had been used as a basis for the decision it would have highlighted, and been more effective on, equity aspects. It focused on prioritized groups and gender throughout and made it an important part of the assessment (see Table CS8.1). Interviewees also stated that if the complementary HIA had been published in time and presented properly to the decision-makers, it would have made it easier to reach a decision earlier and would have underlined the positive health effects of alternative E.

The interviewees also stated that an HIA can be effective in even more dimensions (i.e. cost, decision and administrative effectiveness respectively). However, these were general comments rather than specific to Route 73. The interviewees all appreciate that HIA in accordance with the new public health policy is a good tool for elucidating health aspects and highlighting achievements of social and environmental sustainability for decision-makers. The interviewees had good acceptance of the methods suggested and thought that their use in the future would lead to better informed decisions. This is welcomed by all.

Naturally, interviewees had different opinions and perspectives on effectiveness depending on which organization they represented. This explains their differing answers – for instance, someone representing a local stakeholder would have a different perspective on the project from those representing central agencies. Someone representing an organization dealing with environmental concerns is likely to take another standpoint from those representing the transport sector.

Factors that facilitated or hindered the HIA

In Sweden, several contextual factors play a substantial role in the success of HIA. According to the interviewees, there is a growing awareness of public health in Sweden today due to the policies adopted by the Riksdag and the Government. Public health objectives, the pinpointing of prioritized groups, health determinants and indicators constitute a good framework for conducting HIA in accordance with the new public health policy and represent its prime facilitators. In recent years, central agencies and regional authorities have also been commissioned by the Government to perform HIA in accordance with the new public health policy within their fields.

The interviewees all acknowledged that HIA in accordance with the new public health policy is an excellent tool for assessing health and social sustainability. They also stated that it is important for the quality of the HIA to have a process where competences between and within organizations meet. This creates a culture where it is possible to discuss health issues and social sustainability in other policy sectors.

The interviewees identified the benefits of having an integrated approach towards HIA and making it complementary to, or part of, EIA. This was the case for both the partial HIA of Route 73 and the complementary HIA. HIA should not be a document in isolation but use existing results from the EIA process that consider environmental determinants and complement these with social determinants and the equity perspective. The integration of HIA and EIA is a step towards Sustainability Impact Assessment and it would help to highlight conflicts between the sustainability dimensions.

The interviewees expressed the importance of using experienced and motivated practitioners when performing HIA, as they can be a facilitating factor. It is also important to present the results in an instructive way, making them easy for decision-makers to comprehend and see the differences between the alternatives. This is crucial to success and effectiveness and can facilitate the process.

Several interviewees gave the impression that interests and sectors other than health (apart from accidents and loss of life) play a more important role in decision-making. This was also the case in the construction project on Route 73. Society is taking time to change its perspective on social sustainability and public health. Health issues are far from receiving the same amount of consideration given to other policy sectors. HIA at its core definition is not yet known adequately in society and the new public health policy has yet to be implemented fully. This also explains some of the difficulties encountered in this case study.

Interviewees felt that policy decisions on HIA in accordance with the new public health policy should be taken by politicians at all levels in order to broaden its use, especially at the local level. The Government assigns tasks to central agencies and this can be seen as an important beginning but decisions are needed on all political levels.

One important conclusion from this case study is that HIA in accordance with the new public health policy is felt to be an effective tool for the attainment of social sustainability in Sweden. Partial HIA as a part of EIA is effective but seldom reflects the full intent of the new public health policy. Over the last few years the Swedish Government has taken policy decisions and initiatives to broaden the use of HIA in accordance with the new public health policy, and hopefully this will make it a more common procedure for decision-making. But obstacles must be overcome in order to heighten its profile and ensure it is used on a broader scale.

REFERENCES

European Observatory on Health Systems and Policies (2005). *The effectiveness of health impact assessment. Conceptual framework for task 2, the interviews.* Brussels, European Observatory on Health Systems and Policies.

Government of Sweden (2002). *Mål för folkhälsan [Objectives for public health].* Stockholm, Government of Sweden (Prop. 2002/03:35).

SNIPH (2003). *Sweden's new public health policy. National objectives for Sweden.* Stockholm, Swedish National Institute of Public Health (Report R 2003:45).

SNIPH (2005a). *A guide to health impact assessments. Focusing on social and environmental sustainability.* Stockholm, Swedish National Institute of Public Health (Report R 2005:40).

SNIPH (2005b). *Health impact assessment of a road traffic project. Case-study: Route 73.* Stockholm, Swedish National Institute of Public Health (Report R 2005:42).

Swedish Road Administration (2002). *Environmental impact assessment with supplementary road survey – Route 73 Nynäshamn-Stockholm, Älgviken-Fors section. Consultation documentation March 2002/version 3 UTR 2002:31. Reference number 41540.* Stockholm, Swedish Road Administration.

Citizen involvement in a local HIA: informing decisions on the future of a landfill site in Wales

Eva Elliott, Alison Golby[20] and Gareth Williams

Introduction

This chapter describes a health impact assessment (HIA) of a proposal to remediate a landfill refuse site that had ceased operations. The HIA itself was led by the public health team within the Local Health Board (LHB) who have a responsibility for health and the commissioning of health services within the local authority area. The landfill site ceased to operate in March 2002 and the HIA was conducted from November 2004 to April 2005 by a Remediation Sub-Group. Their remit was to oversee the process of making decisions on how the land, on which the domestic and industrial waste has been deposited, was sealed off and made safe. The results of this HIA fed directly into the final design and implementation plans for the site.

This case study was chosen for a number of reasons. Firstly, HIAs in Wales have been conducted on national policies, local government strategies and programmes as well as small community projects. Strategy and policy development, including health and well-being, have largely been devolved to local government and the bulk of HIAs have been undertaken on this level. For this reason an HIA undertaken within a local authority in Wales was chosen.

---

[20] Alison Golby acted as an observer and adviser for the HIA described in this chapter. Eva Elliott delivered a presentation on HIA at their first stakeholder group meeting and provided comments on the final report that they produced.

Secondly, the HIA has an emphasis on public participation. Since devolution there has been a strong emphasis on the citizen's role in policy-making and enhancing public participation within the new Wales (National Assembly for Wales, 2001; Welsh Assembly Government, 2004). Recent national guidance on the use of HIA (WHIASU, 2004) stresses its value in utilizing the knowledge, views and experiences of local people to inform decisions. This case study exemplifies the way in which the approach has been used in a number of assessments in Wales.

Finally, it was chosen because it was recent enough for key stakeholders to have a clear memory of the process, yet enough time had elapsed for the process to have influenced decisions. This enabled some assessment of how, and in what respects, the HIA may have informed decision-making processes.

Five people were interviewed for this study including those who were involved in leading the HIA, local stakeholders formally involved in the process and an official involved in the Remediation Sub-Group that made the decisions regarding the future of the site. Two respondents were representatives from the statutory sector; the other three were a resident, an elected member and a voluntary sector representative. These three have been referred to as community representatives. To preserve anonymity, where opinion is referred to, the source is attributed to a statutory or community interviewee. Documents associated with the HIA were also reviewed.

This chapter will start with background to the policy context within which HIA is positioned in Wales followed by some contextual details relating to the case study. The chosen HIA will be described according to the methods undertaken, actors involved and its relationship to the decision-making process. The extent to which this has been effective according to the criteria employed by the study is then discussed. Finally the chapter will identify the strengths and weaknesses inherent in the process.

HIA in Wales

Since 1999 certain key powers have been devolved to the National Assembly for Wales. Devolution has provided the country with more control over its own affairs, particularly policy areas including health. Wales has some of the poorest populations in the United Kingdom. The south Wales valleys face significant social and economic hardship, and consequent ill-health, following the demise of the coal and steel industries in those areas. From the outset, the need to improve health and reduce persistent inequalities in the country have been priorities (Welsh Office, 1998; National Assembly for Wales, 2000).

A number of policy and strategy documents have stressed the need for all sectors, levels of government and parts of society to be involved in improving the nation's health (Welsh Assembly Government, 2002; Welsh Assembly Government, 2003). Health Challenge Wales is described as a national focus with "a call to all people and organizations in Wales to work together for a healthier nation". HIA is promoted as a tool to enable organizations to fulfil these responsibilities and to make the link between health and other policy areas (National Assembly for Wales, 1999; Breeze & Hall, 2002). The initial national guidance, *Developing Health Impact Assessment in Wales* (National Assembly for Wales, 2000) led to the implementation of a development programme. This included the creation of the Welsh Health Impact Assessment Support Unit (WHIASU[21]) which was set up to help organizations and groups outside the Welsh Assembly Government to understand and use the approach throughout the country.

Though not a legal requirement, the use of HIA is promoted in national and local policy documents and has a recognized remit within key national and local government bodies. At a national level, the Welsh Local Government Association and the National Public Health Service for Wales support its use. At a local level, HIA is seen as a way of supporting the 22 local authorities and their corresponding LHBs[22] to develop, implement and evaluate statutory local "Health, social care and well-being strategies". In support of this WHIASU produced a guide to HIA (WHIASU, 2004). This was published by the Assembly Government in November 2004, after this HIA commenced.

Background to the HIA in Nant-y-Gwyddon

The Nant-y-Gwyddon landfill site overlooks the Rhondda Valley in south-east Wales, an area with a long history of coal mining and a population struggling with the social and economic legacy of this industry's demise. More recently, the area has become famous in Wales for its waste operations and local residents' angry response to a development which they felt had become a blight on their community.

---

[21] WHIASU is located in the Cardiff Institute of Society Health and Ethics in Cardiff University's School of Social Sciences and in the Wales Centre for Health's base in Wrexham. It is funded through the Wales Centre for Health by the Office of the Chief Medical Officer (OCMO) in the Welsh Assembly Government. The Wales Centre for Health has a statutory remit to develop and maintain arrangements for making information about matters related to the protection and improvement of health available to the public in Wales, to undertake and commission research into such matters and to contribute to the development and provision of training.

[22] The 22 Local Health Boards were set up in April 2003 to replace five Health Authorities. LHBs and local authorities have coterminous boundaries.

The site began waste-disposal operations in 1988; in the mid-1990s their licence was amended to permit the disposal of non-special commercial and industrial waste. The disposal of non-special industrial waste, including calcium sulphate filter cake and the release of hydrogen sulphide which produced noxious odours in the local area, led to public concern about the site's impact on the health of people living in the closest proximity. Persistent complaints such as stress, fatigue, headaches, eye infections, coughs, stuffy noses, dry throat and nausea were reported, which residents linked to exposure to the site (Rhondda Cynon Taff LHB, 2005). More seriously, there was a perceived increase in the number of congenital abnormalities including gastroschisis – a very rare condition where the intestines form outside the abdomen. A study confirmed an increase in birth defects but stressed the difficulties in attributing causality to such clusters (Fielder et al., 2000). This was confirmed in a review of the work undertaken by statutory agencies on the site's effects on the health of the communities. This was organized by the Wales Centre for Health and undertaken by the Agency for Toxic Substances and Disease Registry (ATSDR) in the US Department of Health and Human Services (ATSDR, 2002).

Local people were not persuaded by such scientific scepticism and they set up an action group called RANT (Rhondda Against Nant-y-Gwyddon Tip) to campaign for the closure of the landfill. In March 2002 waste operations were closed down following an independent investigation of a number of broad issues arising from the site (Purchon, 2001). The local authority's Community Waste Forum set up a Remediation Sub-Group comprised of representatives from the relevant statutory and regulatory bodies as well as community representatives, including a member of RANT.[23] The group was charged with the responsibility of identifying the best viable remediation plan, guided by two central principles: that the protection of human health was paramount and that any proposal would be subject to an HIA.

The HIA

The HIA was conducted to demonstrate that the health of local people was being taken into account in the development of plans for the site's future and, by making the process participatory, to involve local people directly in these decisions (Rhondda Cynon Taff LHB, 2005). In addition, the local authority and the LHB were keen to develop HIA. In interviews with statutory representatives they reported that this was an opportunity to test HIAs value

---

[23] The group itself was chaired by an independent facilitator and included a representative from RANT, a member of the local regeneration partnership, the local authority (elected members and officers), the Environmental Agency, the landfill operator, the LHB and an independent medical adviser.

as a tool to improve the way in which the public health implications of such decisions are considered and to develop skills for conducting such assessments.

A strict timetable was imposed to ensure that the process would fit in with decisions on the remediation plans, and a local authority employee was seconded to the LHB to coordinate this work for six months. Statutory interviewees reported that this was to ensure that the skills developed from the HIA would be developed in the organizations involved. Prior to the commencement of the HIA the coordinator attended a 5-day HIA training course delivered by IMPACT. This Liverpool-based organization is one of the first in the United Kingdom to offer intensive training in HIA. The HIA was informed by the Gothenburg consensus (European Centre for Health Policy, 1999) and the process based on guidelines developed by the Health Development Agency in England (HDA, 2002).

Two additional pieces of work were undertaken before the HIA was conducted. Firstly, an investigation of the content of the site including the possible presence of radioactive material – this was found to be negligible. Secondly, the Remediation Sub-Group undertook an exhaustive exercise to identify and appraise all possible remediation options. The option that best satisfied the principles devised to guide the process was known as Containment Plus. This involved the use of a permanent plastic cap, or geomembrane, in conjunction with low-permeability soils to act as a protective barrier. With some re-profiling of the site it was felt that this would improve both stability and the visual impact of the work undertaken (Rhondda Cynon Taff LHB, 2005). Systems to capture, or contain, and dispose of gas and leachate would also be put in place. Although this appraisal process could have been part of the main HIA process, statutory interviewees reported that it was felt to be too technical and intensive to be included. They felt that the Remediation Sub-Group appraisal was inclusive due to the make up of the group, and succeeded in identifying the option that would be most protective of health.

Members of the public were invited to participate in the main HIA in order to provide the maximum opportunity for them to influence the way in which the process was designed and implemented. The HIA highlighted the need to consider equity and to ensure that no particular groups, especially vulnerable groups, were more affected than any other group in the surrounding area (Rhondda Cynon Taff LHB, 2005). Statutory interviewees reported that the HIA was also informed by a broad definition of health and attempted to gauge potential impacts on the broad social, economic and environmental determinants of health.

A stakeholder group was set up to undertake key aspects of the process and to facilitate the partnership approach in order to ensure that the HIA process was participative and inclusive. The Remediation Sub-Group was proposed for this role but it was felt that the process should be linked to but separate from what was effectively the decision-making body. The stakeholder group included a range of people, including RANT and other community representatives affected by the scheme and people with the relevant expertise and knowledge of the remediation process. Meetings were chaired by an independent organization representing the voluntary sector in the local authority area. Four meetings were held and participants played a key role in assessing and prioritizing the evidence that was collected.

Local opinions were gathered from a community exhibition during which a questionnaire was used to gather people's views of the impact of the process, and from 12 focus groups out of 98 invited groups of people in the area. In addition the HIA made use of market research undertaken on behalf of the Remediation Sub-Group which included data from a street survey and in-depth interviews with individuals living near the site. The November 2004 edition of the Nantygwyddon News contained details of the proposal and invited readers to offer their thoughts on the long-term usage of the site. These were fed into the assessment process together with technical reports undertaken on the site itself and any other published research that was relevant to the expected impacts.

Analysis of all the data identified 42 potential impacts on health, reflecting the concern of local residents on how the design and construction of the remediation proposal might affect their health. The stakeholder group used this information to prioritize and judge the likelihood and significance of the impacts and agree on a set of key recommendations. Most of the main recommendations related to ensuring that agreed processes and procedures were adhered to, as well as ensuring that people and animals were prevented from entering the site during construction. An additional recommendation was made to cover the geomembrane cap with spoil from local tips rather than materials from elsewhere which could increase traffic and related hazards.

Dimensions of effectiveness

The key aim of the HIA was to undertake an assessment of the Containment Plus option on behalf of the Remediation Sub-Group, and to contribute to the final design process ensuring that "potential risks to health during and after the remediation scheme implementation are paramount". The process was generally felt to have been successful in meeting stakeholders' expectations of what the HIA could achieve. The HIA was completed within the time frame expected and delivered a set of recommendations on how Containment Plus could be delivered to ensure that the health and well-being of residents were taken into account. These were agreed by the Remediation Sub-Group.

This case study assessed the HIA using the overarching conceptual framework to distinguish different ways in which effectiveness may be understood and addressed. Direct effectiveness refers to examples where (i) the health aspects as addressed by the HIA have been acknowledged in the decision-making process and (ii) the recommendations on health impact have modified a pending decision. A cursory interpretation may conclude that this HIA represents an example of direct health effectiveness since concerns for health were acknowledged in the decision-making process and the recommendations were accepted.

However, decision-making processes are rarely that simple, rational or instrumental. Interviews clearly illuminated the broader politicized arena in which the HIA was played out. The assessment was conducted in response to a long-standing argument between local residents and public agencies and represented an attempt to put the dispute to rest. However, although public involvement was welcome and laudable, it was invited at a relatively uncontroversial moment in the site's history. After all, the subject of the controversy (the tip) had been closed. Respondents themselves agreed that the recommendations were not wholly surprising and, once they had decided to opt for the Containment Plus option, were likely to have been adopted anyway. Indeed the statutory interviewees felt that it gave a mandate to what they were planning and, in this light, could be seen as an example of opportunistic effectiveness. The working definition of this suggests that although the HIA appeared to influence decisions which affect health and well-being it actually justified an existing plan. However, if the setting up of the Remediation Sub-Group and the option-appraisal process (where professional and lay stakeholders identified Containment Plus as the healthiest option) were also considered then it would be reasonable to identify a more direct relationship to the decision-making process.

This raises an important question as to when HIA processes actually began. In this interpretation the HIA process began before the commissioned HIA phase started. Members of the Remediation Sub-Group were themselves deeply concerned about the health impact of any decision that they might make and the principle that the health of local people was paramount shaped the way in which the group operated.

Health effectiveness

Given the history of the site, it is not surprising that the focus was primarily on the environmental impacts on health. In addition, the proposal that local people were asked to consider – the Containment Plus option – was highly technical. Statutory interviewees felt that it was difficult for those directing the process to go beyond explanations of the technical details themselves. In addition, although the HIA used a broad definition of health it was felt to be hard to engage people in discussion of the social and economic determinants. One statutory interviewee argued that although issues around the wider determinants were sometimes articulated they were easier to see in the coding stage of the analysis and harder for residents to identify explicitly as broader impacts on health.

Community effectiveness

All the interviewees felt that an underlying aim of the HIA was to recognize, respond and alleviate residents' anger, anxiety and mistrust that had built up over the previous decade. It was also an opportunity to test the level of concern since, although RANT still existed, it was suspected that since the tip had closed other residents might not continue to share its views regarding the dangers associated with the site.

Although respondents involved in conducting the HIA were disappointed with the lack of representation of particular groups, essentially men and young people, they felt that everything had been done to communicate with local people and all residents, through a variety of mechanisms, were given an opportunity to present their views. Respondents from the statutory agencies viewed it as a chance to close a chapter in the site's history and confirm that the majority of local residents no longer appeared to share the views of RANT. Respondents interpreted the lack of interest from some groups, who were invited to participate but chose not to, as an indication that most residents had no concerns about possible health risks from the Containment Plus option. However, although RANT representatives participated in a focus group, and had representation on the stakeholder group and the Remediation Sub-Group, they withdrew halfway through the process and continued to voice concerns about the site. No member of RANT was interviewed for this case study.

In addition, community involvement impacted on two additional specific options linked to the implementation of the remediation plans that were not resolved by the Remediation Sub-Group. The first related to power generation and whether the power captured and generated from the site could be utilized. The second related to undertaking further possible bioremediation of the site. One statutory representative interviewed said that the views of the community were considered to be valid and very useful, particularly a number of clearly articulated concerns about the possible impacts of the bioremediation process.

These views impacted directly on more recent decisions to proceed with plans to use power generated from the site but not for further bioremediation.

All interviewees felt that the HIA had been an effective method of engaging with local people, despite the small numbers of men and young people involved. This HIA revealed a key finding – local people felt that the HIA process had been the first time that the statutory agencies had explained properly what was planned for the site. However, one community representative felt that there was not enough attention to the use of the site once construction was completed, and that the local community may have useful views to contribute to this aspect of the site's future.

Equity effectiveness

The team guiding the HIA deliberately set out to assess the distribution of the effects on different population groups and to ensure that vulnerable groups were not disadvantaged by the scheme. However, the variation of impacts on different groups was not marked enough to filter through into the recommendations. This may be partly attributable to the lack of representation from some groups. Although the HIA team attempted to canvass a diverse range of opinion, there was a distinct lack of representation in younger age groups and nearly twice as many women as men participated. However, one community respondent argued that younger groups may not have felt the site to be an issue and therefore were not interested in participating. Attempts were made to ensure that attendance at focus groups was not hindered by access problems so time, place and child care responsibilities were unlikely to be issues.

Other dimensions of effectiveness

Asked about other ways in which the HIA could be considered effective, a statutory representative reported that although financial costs had been high, the process itself had been cost-effective. Over the last few years significant resources have been invested in studies responding to residents' concerns about the site. It has also been subject to a great deal of political controversy. As a result of the HIA, and having taken stock of the views of local people, decisions on the need for further public health investigations of the site could be made on the basis of more robust evidence of the current and ongoing concerns of different stakeholders. In addition the HIA was reported to have had an organizational impact by investing in staff skills which could be utilized in future assessments. Finally, statutory interviewees reported its effectiveness in ensuring that decision-makers were confident that they could now close an issue that had been in the public eye for many years.

Facilitating and inhibiting factors

In this particular HIA there was no doubt that the process would influence decisions because the Remediation Sub-Group had agreed that their decisions would be guided by its recommendations. However, it is unlikely that the HIA would have taken place without key individuals who championed the process at particular times.

In the first instance the Head of Public Protection, a local authority officer, called for the HIA to be undertaken. This was strongly supported by the Acting Director of Public Health from the LHB. The report acknowledged the Welsh Assembly Government's support for HIA so national endorsement for the process may have helped. In addition, local authority boundaries are now coterminous with those of the new LHBs and this may have contributed to these statutory organizations' willingness, and capacity, to collaborate on this project for mutual benefit. The HIA was conducted on behalf of the Remediation Sub-Group which ensured that the process was timed to synchronize with decisions on the remediation process, and feedback of the recommendations was provided at the optimum time. The HIA coordinator was line-managed by the Acting Public Health Director from the LHB, a member of the Sub-Group. This ensured tight project management of the process.

The effectiveness of the process was attributable to a number of factors. Firstly, community and statutory interviewees recognized the LHB's role as the HIA's lead organization. It was reported that residents blamed the local authority for the handling of the site, but this deeply ingrained sense of mistrust was not directed at the LHB which was felt to be an honest broker in this venture. This may also have contributed to a perceived distancing from the politics of the site which had been a controversial and highly visible issue for political parties associated with the decisions of the local authority at different periods in its history. One community respondent highlighted that the LHB's lead forged an ethos of trust from the outset.

The conduct of stakeholder meetings may have been eased by the appointment of an independent chairperson. Ground rules regarding respect for different views were laid down at the very first meeting. However, the chairperson had been involved in another HIA where conflicts of views were expressed with heightened emotions, producing an uneasy process to manage. In the end, remediation plans for the site did not appear to be controversial but were seen as broadly positive. It may be that these factors facilitated the mutual support and collaboration that community and statutory representatives reported to be evident throughout most aspects of the HIA process.

Conclusion

Although it is not possible to identify a typical HIA in Wales and there is no legal requirement to conduct one at any level of government, there is a push to develop a public health culture. The current national focus for health, *Health Challenge Wales*, urges all levels of government, the media, all sectors and members of the public to recognize their own roles in health improvement. A more tangible lever is the statutory duty of all local authorities to work with LHBs to develop health, social care and well-being strategies. Current guidance for these stresses the value of HIA and provides the impetus to conduct assessments in Wales.

Possibly the greatest facilitator for ensuring that the HIA informed the decision-making in this case was the decision-makers own commitment to the process. This required a certain degree of risk as the arm's-length approach taken by the Remediation Sub-Group and commitment to a participative approach meant that recommendations could have challenged directly the views of the statutory agencies. However, they appreciated the potential value of community engagement in producing healthy outcomes and the process itself was felt to be beneficial. In this case the HIA was felt to have informed local people of plans that would affect their lives and helped to forge a relationship of trust between the community and the statutory agencies.

REFERENCES

ATSDR (2002). *Public health investigations at the Nant-y-Gwyddon landfill site, Gelli, Rhondda Cynon Taff: an evaluation of the environmental health assessment process.* Atlanta, United States Department of Health and Human Services.

Breeze C, Hall R (2002). *Health impact assessment in government policy making: developments in Wales.* Copenhagen, European Centre for Health Policy, WHO Regional Office for Europe (Policy Learning Curve Series, No.6 – May).

European Centre for Health Policy (1999). *Health impact assessment: main concepts and suggested approach. Gothenburg consensus paper.* Brussels, WHO Regional Office for Europe.

Fielder HMP, et al. (2000). Assessment of impact on health of residents living near the Nant-y-Gwyddon landfill site: retrospective analysis. *British Medical Journal,* 320:19–23.

HDA (2002). *Introducing health impact assessment (HIA): informing the decision-making process.* London, Health Development Agency.

National Assembly for Wales (1999). *Developing health impact assessment in Wales: better health better Wales.* Cardiff, National Assembly for Wales (http://new.wales.gov.uk/topics/health/improvement/communities/health-impact/publications/developing/?lang=en, accessed 20 March 2007).

National Assembly for Wales (2000). *Better Wales: strategic plan of the National Assembly for Wales.* Cardiff, National Assembly for Wales.

National Assembly for Wales (2001). *Improving health in Wales: a plan for the NHS with its partners.* Cardiff, National Assembly for Wales.

Purchon DP (2001). *Independent investigation of Nant-y-Gwyddon landfill site: investigator's report to the National Assembly for Wales Environment and Planning and Transport Committee.* Cardiff, National Assembly for Wales.

Rhondda Cynon Taff LHB (2005). *The future of Nant-y-Gwyddon: a health impact assessment of the remediation proposals for the Nant-y-Gwyddon landfill site.* Treforest, Rhondda Cynon Taff Local Health Board.

Welsh Assembly Government (2002). *Well-being in Wales: a consultation document.* Cardiff, Welsh Assembly Government.

Welsh Assembly Government (2003). *Wales: a better country: the strategic agenda of the Welsh Assembly Government (September).* Cardiff, Welsh Assembly Government.

Welsh Assembly Government (2004). *Making the connection: delivering better services in Wales.* Cardiff, Welsh Assembly Government.

Welsh Health Impact Assessment Support Unit (WHIASU) (2004). *Improving health and reducing inequalities: a practical guide to health impact assessment.* Cardiff, Welsh Assembly Government.

Welsh Office (1998). *Better health better Wales: a consultation paper.* Cardiff, Welsh Office.

Part IV
The Effectiveness of Integrating Health in Other Impact Assessments: Case Studies

A participative social impact assessment at the local level: supporting the land-use planning process in Finland

Kirsi Nelimarkka, Tapani Kauppinen and Kerttu Perttilä

Introduction

In Finland, assessing the impact of plans is regulated by law. Section 9 of the Land Use and Building Act states:

> Plans must be founded on adequate studies and reports. When a plan is drawn up, the environmental impact of implementing the plan, including socioeconomic, social, cultural and other impacts, must be assessed to the necessary extent. Such an assessment must cover the entire area in which the plan may be expected to have a material impact.

This chapter studies the effectiveness of health impact assessment (HIA). In the context of planning, health impacts and determinants are often combined with social impacts, for which this study will employ the term Social Impact Assessment (SIA). The focus of the analysis was on areas and administrative sectors where impact assessment is already an embedded practice. In order to identify an effective impact assessment, the assessment reports were analysed carefully and the selection discussed with local contacts. On the basis of this preparatory work the SIA of the Korteniitty (situated in the city of Jyväskylä) local detailed plan was selected for the study.

This assessment is prospective, includes stakeholder involvement and community participation and was finalized quite recently. The City of Jyväskylä has a long tradition in the development of planning-related SIA. The Korteniitty SIA has been improved using new tools and processes, for the most part through use of their own resources and cooperation between the planners and representatives of the Centre for Social and Health Services.

The study is based on interviews with 5 interviewees: officials, politicians and residents who took part in the Korteniitty planning process. Also, documents related to the plan's preparation and SIA, such as SIA reports, the plan commentary and the reports of the proceedings of the city council are employed in the study.

This chapter begins with the background of the Korteniitty local detailed plan and its assessment process. This is followed by the aims of the SIA and its effectiveness from the point of view of health, equity and community. The next section contains more detail about the SIA process and context, while the conclusions examine the positive and negative factors bearing on the effectiveness of SIA.

Detailed local plan for Korteniitty

The term SIA was used to describe the Korteniitty assessment process because it is an established term in land-use planning. SIA is partly synonymous with HIA according to a broad definition of health, since both take account of physical, psychological and social dimensions. In connection with the Korteniitty plan, however, the impacts on health were viewed in terms of safety in transporting oneself from one place to another and as road traffic-related disadvantages, according to a narrower definition of health. Psychological and social dimensions were covered in the assessment of social impacts. Although determinants of health (Whitehead & Dahlgren, 1991), such as living conditions and the availability of services, are included as elements in SIA they are not referred to as such.

The detailed local plan for Korteniitty covers the city of Jyväskylä (83 000 residents). Jyväskylä's Planning Office was responsible for the planning of the proposed residential area 2.5 km north-west of Jyväskylä city centre. The site of Korteniitty is located within the Kortepohja residential area (6700 residents) and Rautpohjanlahti, which consists mainly of vacant farmland, recreational land and forest (Jyväskylän kaupunki, 2005a).

The aim of the Korteniitty plan was to complement the residential construction of Kortepohja with low and dense construction situated between the blocks of

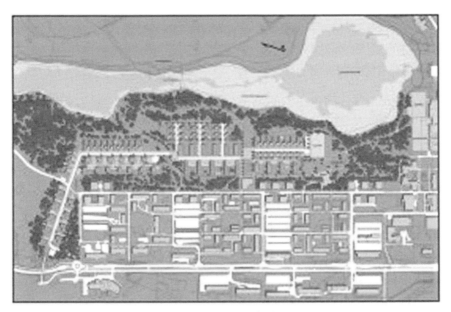

Figure CS10.1 *View from Korteniitty second draft plan*

flats and individual houses (Figure CS10.1). According to the plan, the permitted building volume is 35 000 km², which means 700 new residents. The planned area is 53 hectares. (Jyväskylän kaupunki, 2003; Jyväskylän kaupunki, 2005a).

The Korteniitty area had been in the city's planning programme for a long time before planning began. The area's construction had been studied as part of a local master plan and in preliminary city plan studies. Having encountered major opposition the planning process was interrupted in the 1990s. The city restarted planning in October 2001, a general draft plan was completed during the autumn of 2002 and the first draft plan was made publicly available in February 2003. In the light of feedback received, it was decided to draw up a revised draft plan by the end of 2003. It was available for public inspection in January 2004 (Jyväskylän kaupunki, 2005a) In autumn 2005, the Korteniitty proposal was made available for public inspection for a month. The City Council approved the plan at its meeting in November 2005 (Jyväskylän kaupunki, 2005b).

The alternatives included in the plan's preparation mainly concerned traffic planning in Korteniitty (Jyväskylän kaupunki, 2005a). Since the plan had certain, well-defined objectives, the option of taking no action (the so-called zero option) was not considered feasible. The assessment of health impacts concentrated on the alleviation of adverse effects. According to the interviewees, the following health impacts or determinants were predominant in the impact assessment: recreation, a pleasant environment, safe communications and the adverse effects of traffic.

For the impact assessment of the plan, the Planning Office collaborated with local actors in Kortepohja. The area's social and health service officials and the school held separate meetings regarding the Kortepohja plans between December 2001 and April 2002. Following this, the Korteniitty plan and its SIA were discussed in the meetings of the Kortepohja local liaison committee in December 2002 and November 2003 (Mäkäräinen, 2005). The liaison committee had representatives from both of Kortepohja's day-care centres, the Torpanperä activity centre, Kortepohja residents' association and the local A guild. The area's residents were also heard in public meetings and elsewhere (Mäkäräinen, 2003).

Interviewees' opinions regarding the aims of the Korteniitty SIA can be summarized into five issues:

1 *Fulfil the legal obligations* for the assessment, since impact assessment is required by law in conjunction with planning.
2 Support the planning of the area and the planning process by *generating information* on the effects on the need and capacity of the service and community infrastructure (for example, the area's suitability for further construction; how to make it function well in social terms, and attractive and sustainable in relation to the old Kortepohja; what kinds of changes in service needs should be expected).
3 *Assist in including residents' views on planning and handling conflicts.* Since there was foreseeable opposition to the planning process, the consultation and SIA needed a strong focus.
4 *Consult various citizen groups* (for example, children and young people).
5 *Ensure fluent progress and general acceptance of the plan.* One interviewee wondered whether or not the SIA was acting as a justification for the whole project, claiming that SIA often tries to persuade objectors that no adverse effects will result from the plan. The same interviewee remarked that the assessment was not objective, as the planner and assessor was the same person.

Those interviewed felt that these goals were met, especially in terms of consultation and conflict management. Consultation was constructive and the officials worked in an open and attentive manner. Aspects that caused the most discontent were dropped from the plan which was modified according to residents' opinions. The assessment also met the legal requirements. It produced adequate information for the planning of services, and helped weigh up different points of view. Realization of the SIA's substantial targets, such as social functioning in the area, remains to be seen.

The interviewees felt that the assessment served the interests of the various groups with varying success. Children and families were taken into account; the interests of the elderly received least attention (see section on equity effectiveness).

Dimensions of effectiveness

According to the interviewees, the SIA's direct effects on the plan were difficult to distinguish. However, they remarked that the SIA supported discussion, planning and decision-making; and the perspectives it offered helped to formulate arguments for the decisions made, while providing the residents with information. The SIA strengthened and expedited the planning process while supporting consultation and the analysis of opinion.

The plan report summary (Jyväskylän kaupunki, 2005a) mentions how the impact assessment influenced the planning decisions.

> Based on the impact assessment, it was evident that the SIA had the following influences: defining the location and nature of the bridges crossing Rautpohjanlahti, defining the boundaries and nature of the green spaces and recreational areas, checking the locations of the pathways in the parks and marking part of the playground as a conservation area due to its trees, allocating the southern playground a possible maintenance building and adding two possible construction areas to the plan in order to provide a day-care centre or other social and health services. Additionally, various city area plans were used to create building diversity.

One interviewee stated – contrary to general opinion – that the SIA had no effect on the planning decisions since their impacts were known and the SIA provided no general information. This person felt that the decisions were influenced by the proactivity of the residents and politicians.

Health effectiveness

Interviewees had various views of the SIA's effectiveness on health. The most common perception was that the plan was likely to have minor health impacts so health was a minor theme in the assessment, rated as general in terms of health effectiveness.

In the Korteniitty SIA, health issues were included in the discussions through the health determinants. One interviewee pointed out that health issues emerged indirectly, e.g. in discussions about recreational areas, sports facilities, traffic-planning and access for those with disabilities. Although health aspects were not among the most important justifications behind the planning decisions, interviewees mentioned that these aspects comprised one argument supporting some of the decisions. For instance, direct health effectiveness can be seen in that certain traffic-planning arrangements were changed due to noise and safety implications. These solutions aimed to diminish the weaknesses and adverse effects of the plan.

One interviewee stated that health effectiveness was opportunistic, because health aspects acted partly as arguments to support ready-made decisions. Another interviewee suggested that residents also aimed to achieve health effectiveness based on traffic-planning – certain solutions were rejected on the grounds of safety since they would have increased traffic volumes near homes. The interviewee stated that in reality the traffic flow would be relocated not removed. At the same time, the increasing distance between new residents and services created negative effects in the form of increased traffic emissions and decreased availability and sustainability of services.

Equity effectiveness

The interviewees perceived equity from the perspective of the various social groups involved. Many families with children live in the area and therefore the children's point of view was highlighted in the process. The SIA had direct equity effectiveness as the plan was modified and adjusted accordingly. For example, preserving the playground at its present size and expanding the school playing field when it was relocated, thus improving recreational possibilities in the Kortepohja area. In addition, the safety of children's recreational activities was discussed.

At the planning stage preceding land use, planning decisions concerning the types of houses and apartments and forms of occupancy affect the future socioeconomic structure of the resident population. Some interviewees felt that the Korteniitty local detailed plan did not change the area's socioeconomic structure. As Kortepohja is a middle-class, private housing area, the new plan will attract more middle-class residents and the plan's equity consequences (with regard to different income categories, for instance) will be negligible, giving the SIA general effectiveness.

Those interviewed remarked that certain social groups, such as the elderly and those with mobility problems, were not considered adequately in the plan. People who had lived in the area would have liked to move back, provided that apartments suitable for older people were built. The initial draft plan included lift-equipped housing for the elderly near the pedestrian walkway, close to local services; other houses in the planned area were likely to be low enough not to warrant lifts and therefore were unsuitable for elderly people. Kortepohja residents were against the building of high, lift-equipped housing for cultural and historical reasons since such housing would have changed the look of the old area too radically. According to interviewees, another motive for protesting against lift-equipped housing may have been the loss of the lake view. Lift-equipped housing was removed from the draft plan due to this opposition. Multi-level apartments are unsuitable for people with mobility problems and the lack of proper housing will affect the nature of the Korteniitty area and dictate the types of possible residents. Only the planner defended the interests of elderly people as no suitable expert participated actively in the assessment process. Simultaneously, the position of older people is an example of general effectiveness, since their viewpoints were discussed but not taken into account by the final plan because of the opposition.

There was conflict between present and future residents as naturally they had very different interests regarding the Korteniitty area. One interviewee remarked that current residents had an advantage over future ones who, typically, were represented by the planner alone.

One interviewee mentioned that equity bore no direct influence on the decisions made, since single issues are often subsumed in the general spectrum of issues during planning.

Community effectiveness

According to the interviewees, the Korteniitty SIA was most effective in taking account of the community viewpoint. The majority felt that direct community effectiveness was realized: residents were active and their participation affecting the planning decisions, although this process was not necessarily represented in the arguments for the decisions.

Residents were concerned about safe communications, the number of recreational areas and the preservation of fields, opportunities for physical and outdoor activities and playgrounds. They also suggested a lower permitted building volume and a smaller number of buildings, and it proved possible to have an impact in these respects. Some of the southern blocks opposed by the residents were removed from the plan. According to the interviewees, public opinion was also instrumental in changing road alignments, playing fields, construction schedules and individual elements in the plan (for example, guaranteeing privacy to small plots). The possibilities for playing sports such as soccer and ice hockey were ensured by the expansion of the Kortepohja School field, and the preservation of the southern Kortepohja field as the area's public recreation site.

The interviews revealed that local actors and authorities saw such effectiveness as being due to the actors' inclusion in the assessment process. The local liaison committee acted as an effective channel of communication and participation, for example, the interests of families with children were represented through the committee, ensuring direct community effectiveness. One interviewee referred to the low level of activity of some local authorities, probably being due to rapid staff turnover and centralized management.

One interviewee cited evidence of opportunistic community effectiveness, suggesting that the plan might have been stripped down even without the residents' feedback. The interviewee wondered whether the draft plan had been made too elaborate on purpose, allowing Kortepohja residents to influence it to the point where the permitted building volume would be the amount desired by the planners.

Organizational effectiveness

The SIA also demonstrated organizational effectiveness, the plan being drawn up according to the impact assessment model developed by the City of Jyväskylä. Planning officials gained experience of the functionality of the SIA form, which helped the Planning Office in providing general instructions for the planning process. Furthermore, the SIA activated cooperation and enhanced communication between various administrative areas, increasing the ability to take action and reach agreements, and made the actors commit to the planning process.

The SIA also opened discussions on future needs and possibilities in different administrative areas. The local liaison committee acted as an information channel for the various administrative areas which were then able to plan their own actions and organize services more effectively. Local actors got to know each other better and lowered the threshold for informal cooperation and mutual consultation between the authorities.

SIA as a collaboration process

The Korteniitty SIA began at the same time as the plan, spring 2002, and integrated with its design process. The assessment was handled at various meetings and in negotiations along the way (Figure CS10.2). The impact assessment had seven phases (Mäkäräinen, 2003):

1 Discovering needs and planning the assessment
2 Acquiring basic information
3 Identifying and defining impacts
4 Assessing impacts

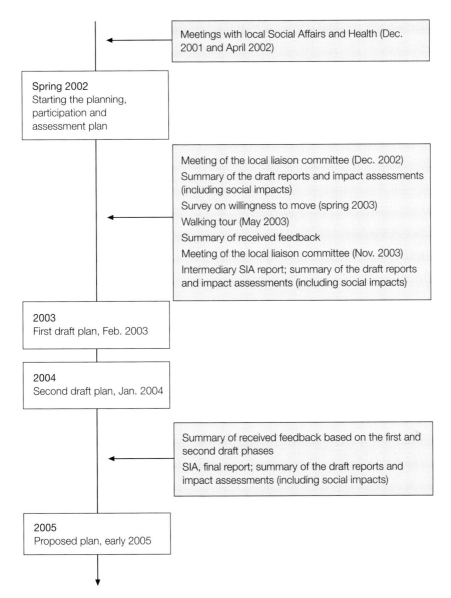

Figure CS10.2 *Main phases of the Korteniitty SIA*

5 Presenting impacts as part of a draft or plan commentary
6 Examining the adequacy of the assessment
7 Assessment follow-up.

The assessment was based on the existing reports, other preparatory materials and additional clarifications made during the planning process. The plan's impacts were identified and their significance considered with the aid of the checklist available in the Planning Office's planning process guide. Plan assessment materials were produced in various meetings as part of the feedback received during the public inspection period. In addition, information on impacts was obtained from plan-related discussion events, a walking tour involving local actors, a survey and discussions with the local liaison committee (Jyväskylän kaupunki, 2005a; Mäkäräinen, 2003; Mäkäräinen, 2005).

The first and second drafting phase each had separate summaries to present the impact assessment situation and key effects. The plan commentary included key social impacts and a summary, similar to those prepared in earlier phases, and was drawn up on the impact assessment. There was also a final report on the social impacts (Jyväskylän kaupunki, 2005a; Mäkäräinen, 2003; Mäkäräinen, 2005).

From resistance to mutual understanding

The Kortepohja area has a strong local identity and residents were active from the very beginning of the planning process through channels including the residents' association. Some town councillors also lived in the area.

One interviewee recounted how the planning process was launched under unfavourable circumstances. The Planning Office did not have time to announce that planning had begun, and the likely additional construction was publicized in the local paper following a tip-off from residents. For this reason, the Planning Office was viewed as secretive and citizens feared that officials would disregard their wishes.

In the initial phase, the Planning Office communicated mainly with officials, consulting residents only as the plan took shape. One interviewee stated that residents initially criticized the SIA as being too centred on the service structure and officials' standpoint. Residents would have wanted to take part in the definition of the impacts, as they felt that their understanding of the adverse effects was better than that of the officials. Residents had little faith that their views would be considered.

The initial draft plan received a significant amount of publicity and opposition, one interviewee remarking that the plan had all the makings of a broader conflict. The residents' association urged people to contribute and write responses and comments. Residents held their own discussion meetings and were active at general public meetings. They also contacted the planner directly, for example, sending petitions and children's drawings.

Following the initial draft plan, the situation settled down. One interviewee thought this might have been because the plan was modified according to residents' viewpoints, and residents were growing accustomed to the idea of the development or giving up hope. Some residents saw positive sides to the new construction from the beginning. Although the schools and day-care centres are full at the moment, Kortepohja's population is ageing and there is a long-term threat of losing services unless there is new construction. Despite their initial opposition, the community was satisfied with the end result. The local detailed plan received only one complaint, and even that was resolved through negotiation.

Law as the starting point, the city as the developer

Since the law presupposes an impact assessment when planning land use, the concomitant legal requirements formed the framework for the SIA. The planner from the Planning Office and SIA project worker were responsible for the assessment's kick-off, practicalities and progress. The assessment model developed by the SIA project worker, together with the assessment form, was used in the Korteniitty SIA; the City of Jyväskylä defrayed the assessment costs.

The SIA did not have an official steering group but the plan's project group performed this function. The group comprised representatives from the Planning Office (taking the lead), Land Division Department, Street and Park Maintenance, Water Supply and Distribution, Centre for Social and Health Services, Housing Office and Centre for Physical Recreation Services. At the start, the plan was presented a few times to the executive team of the Centre for Social and Health Services, western area.

The Planning Office employed discussion-based, proactive steering processes, such as internal guidance, negotiations between the various parties, reviews and hearings. Many interviewees remarked that the planner and SIA project worker had an open and attentive approach, although the Planning Office had yet to become wholeheartedly proactive.

The Land Use and Building Act (132/1999) presupposes certain consultative and participative proceedings during the various stages of the planning process. At the same time the law requires that such arrangements and the impact assessment be properly scheduled and that there is a genuine opportunity to influence matters (Figure CS10.3). In the Korteniitty planning process, the participative proceedings exceeded the minimum level required by law, due partly to the enthusiasm aroused by the development work and partly to the great challenges posed by the planning project. It is not known why organizations did not participate proactively in the SIA but one interviewee cited the area's location outside the city centre as a possible reason.

Politicians' role in the assessment divided opinion. Some felt that political participation in the SIA was low-key, while the interviews in general indicated that politicians had the residents' interests at heart. The Green League has a strong foothold on the Planning Board, as well as in Korteniitty. This is a

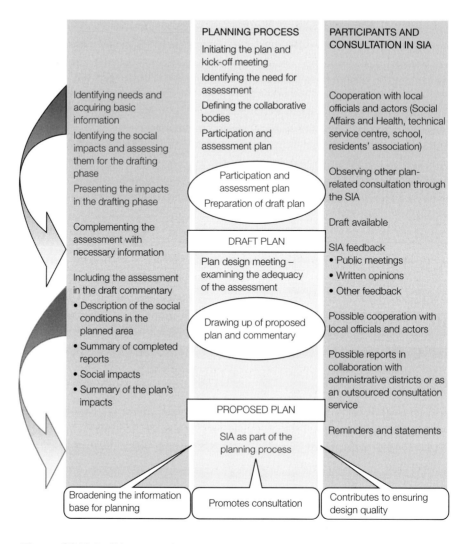

The following text labels appear within the figure:

PLANNING PROCESS

Initiating the plan and kick-off meeting

Identifying the need for assessment

Defining the collaborative bodies

Participation and assessment plan

Participation and assessment plan
Preparation of draft plan

DRAFT PLAN

Plan design meeting – examining the adequacy of the assessment

Drawing up of proposed plan and commentary

PROPOSED PLAN

SIA as part of the planning process

PARTICIPANTS AND CONSULTATION IN SIA

Cooperation with local officials and actors (Social Affairs and Health, technical service centre, school, residents' association)

Observing other plan-related consultation through the SIA

Draft available

SIA feedback
• Public meetings
• Written opinions
• Other feedback

Possible cooperation with local officials and actors

Possible reports in collaboration with administrative districts or as an outsourced consultation service

Reminders and statements

Identifying needs and acquiring basic information

Identifying the social impacts and assessing them for the drafting phase

Presenting the impacts in the drafting phase

Complementing the assessment with necessary information

Including the assessment in the draft commentary
• Description of the social conditions in the planned area
• Summary of completed reports
• Social impacts
• Summary of the plan's impacts

Broadening the information base for planning

Promotes consultation

Contributes to ensuring design quality

Figure CS10.3 *SIA as part of the planning process in Jyväskylä*

political party that places emphasis on the role of civil society, having its roots in nature and environment protection. Parliamentary elections coincided with the draft plan and meeting for the general public; local politicians responded with speeches favourable to residents in an attempt to win political capital. In addition, politicians contacted the planners, for example, via e-mail.

Although the Korteniitty development plan became a political issue, the SIA did not incite any political conflicts. Those interviewed stated that since the impact assessment was integrated with the planning process, politicians did not treat the assessment as a distinct issue during committee meetings on the plans. Politicians also lacked the time to give detailed consideration to the reports and SIA. Impacts were barely discussed during committee meetings, the lion's share of attention going to changes in the plan and reactions to feedback but certainly the SIA made politicians more aware of the impacts.

No strong culture has developed to take account of public health in planning, although health issues are investigated to a certain extent during planning (e.g. through factors with an impact on health). According to the interviewees, public health is taken into account in terms of minimizing adverse effects as required by law. Noise pollution is often discussed during planning, but this was irrelevant to Korteniitty since no major roads were planned. One interviewee felt that politicians tend to ignore public health-related planning issues, planners having insufficient means to influence such issues despite awareness of them. One person claimed that it was possible to have an impact on public health through planning, by creating the necessary conditions for recreational sporting activities or social interaction, although no plan can oblige residents to behave in a certain way.

Conclusion

The preparation and application of the SIA for the Korteniitty local detailed plan progressed as integrated processes. This makes it difficult to study SIA effectiveness as it is difficult to ascertain whether changes to the plans were due to impact assessment. When assessment forms an integral part of other design aspects it has the best chance of influencing decisions. Often SIA already plays a role in minor and major choices made during the planning phase, and not solely in the final plan.

This study reveals the SIA's impact on the Korteniitty local detailed plan and its effect on planning decisions. It had direct effectiveness especially in the community aspect; health and equity effectiveness were mainly direct or general. The most important factors explaining the effectiveness of the SIA are related to processes and contextual factors, such as the local culture and practices in SIA, the cooperation networks supporting the SIA, and community dynamics.

Sustained SIA development as practised by the City of Jyväskylä has created a permanent culture in city planning, which views advance impact assessment favourably. This has provided the planner with concrete tools to help in such assessments.

Effectiveness is linked strongly to the way in which individual officials work and their attitudes. In Korteniitty, initial doubts cleared and gave way to feelings of trust and genuine consideration of the community viewpoint, owing to a discussion-based approach. A clear indication of this is the low number of complaints received about the plan.

In Jyväskylä, collaborative relationships created during the development work (for instance, with the Centre for Social and Health Services) ensured that the assessment included information on different social groups and their needs. The SIA's use of existing structures, such as the long-standing activities of the Kortepohja local liaison committee, helped to bring local, experience-based information into the assessment. A new group would have needed time for members to get to know one another and the group's working methods, and would have had fewer opportunities to influence decision-making.

Kortepohja's active residents also played a key role with respect to local factors. In addition to a strong local identity, they knew and utilized their own opportunities and rights to contribute to the planning process. The residents' association was able to have more impact than a single resident working alone. It can be said that the Korteniitty SIA process supported the empowerment of a community where the activity of local residents was already high. The effectiveness of SIA could be increased, especially in connection with the equity aspect, by galvanizing various social groups and officials to participate in the assessment process. The equity aspect can also be supported by the collection and analysis of information on different population groups in the assessment process.

Often, assessing health impacts means the mere identification of environmental risks and the alleviation of adverse effects. SIAs take account of factors included in a broader definition of health but seldom refer to them as health issues. Discussion of the cumulative impact of various factors on human health and well-being is needed to bring the health aspect to the fore in the planning process. In addition to being able to identify the impacts of a decision on the determinants of health, it is necessary to be able to draw health conclusions concerning the decision.

REFERENCES

Jyväskylän kaupunki [City of Jyväskylä] (2003). *Osallistumis- ja arviointisuunnitelma. Korteniitty. [Participation and assessment plan. Korteniitty].* Kaavatunnus [Plan number] 17:085. Päiväys [Date] 21.11.2003. Jyväskylä, Jyväskylän kaupunki [City of Jyväskylä] (http://www. jyvaskyla.fi/kaavoitus/pdf/KN_oas.pdf, accessed 9 January 2006).

Jyväskylän kaupunki [City of Jyväskylä] (2005a). *Asemakaavan selostus. Korteniitty [Commentary for local detailed plan. Korteniitty].* Kaavatunnus [Plan number] 17:085. Päiväys [Date] 31.5.2005. Jyväskylä, Jyväskylän kaupunki [City of Jyväskylä] (http://www.jyvaskyla.fi/kaavoitus/ pdf/selostus_Korteniitty.pdf, accessed 9 January 2006).

Jyväskylän kaupunki [City of Jyväskylä] (2005b). *Kaupunginvaltuuston kokouspöytäkirja, 14 Marraskuuta 2005, §183 [Minutes of the city council meeting, 14 November 2005, 183]* (http://www.jyvaskyla.fi/paatos/ kv/2005/14111800.1/htmtxt183.htm, accessed 9 January 2006).

Maankäyttö- ja rakennuslaki 132/1999. [Land Use and Building Act 132/1999]. Suomen säädöskokoelma [Statutes of Finland]. Helsinki, Oy Edita Ab.

Mäkäräinen J (2003). *Askel kohti ihmistä. Kaavoituksen sosiaalisten vaikutusten arviointia kehittäneen Sva-projektin loppuraportti [A step towards humanity. Final report in the SIA development project].* Jyväskylän sosiaali- ja terveyspalvelukeskuksen julkaisuja 1/2003. Jyväskylä, Jyväskylän kaupungin sosiaali- ja terveyspalvelukeskus & Kaupunkisuunnittelutoimisto [The Centre for Social and Health Services & Jyväskylä's Planning Office].

Mäkäräinen J (2005). *Sosiaalinen eheys yhdyskuntasuunnittelussa. Kokemuksia Jyväskylän kaupunkiseudulta [Social unity in community planning. Experiences from the Jyväskylä urban area].* Suomen ympäristö 798. Ympäristöministeriö [Ministry of the Environment]. Helsinki, Edita Prima Oy.

Whitehead M, Dahlgren G (1991). What can we do about inequalities in health? *Lancet,* 338:1059–1063.

Case study 11

The controversial Berlin Brandenburg International Airport: time- and resource-consuming efforts concerning health within planning approval in Germany

Rudolf Welteke, Thomas Classen, Odile Mekel and Rainer Fehr

Introduction

This chapter presents the health aspects of a typical German planning process. It deals with expected health consequences while following the instructions and instruments defined by the environmental impact assessment (EIA) regulation and the specific German regulated procedure *Planfeststellungsverfahren* (project approval procedure due to technical legislation) which are carried out when large projects with a high degree of complexity are planned. The focus for this case study is the assessment of noise pollution effects, which have been thoroughly examined by several experts during the planning procedure and during the proceedings in the Supreme Court of Law.

This chapter includes a health impact assessment (HIA)-related analysis of different categories of population effects caused by the Berlin Brandenburg International (BBI) project, such as the health, social and community implications of the new airport. The positive and negative aspects of the

German approach for dealing with these types of projects are discussed, as well as HIA-related demands. The information is based on a series of five detailed interviews conducted with employees and functional executives involved directly in the planning process. The interviews took place between May and June 2006. Public agencies and parties responsible for the BBI and airport opponents joined the interviews. In addition, contacts were made with some state ministries. Additional information refers to publications.[24] The BBI project was chosen from a German HIA sample collection compiled in 2005. The selection criteria included topicality; significance of the project; scope of the project; relevance to health; the procedure's model-like qualities; and public involvement and access to materials and information.

HIA-related activities were driven by official actors, the participation of affected communities and, last but not least, a legal decision. The majority of the results focused on adjusting several dimensions of the planning process in favour of better human health protection. The main development leading to improved noise protection was realized by the court decision on the new BBI airport, including a complete night-flight ban between 24:00 and 05:00, and limited air traffic between 05:00 and 06:00, and between 22:00 and 24:00. As a consequence, the HIA activities showed a certain degree of effectiveness according to health and community dimensions. However, analysis of the entire process pointed to a serious lack of efficiency for the BBI planning procedures, especially when assessing future health issues.

Profiling the BBI airport HIA

The BBI planning process

The BBI project was designed to create a modern, full-size international airport close to Berlin following two key events – the reunification of Germany in 1990 and the decision to move the federal capital from Bonn to Berlin in 1991. The States of Berlin and Brandenburg and the Federal Republic of Germany came to an agreement in 1991 that an international large-scale single airport should replace the existing three inner-city or suburban airports of Tempelhof, Tegel and Schönefeld.

The planning process for the large-scale BBI airport started in 1992 as part of the regional planning procedure in the state of Brandenburg and was completed temporarily in 1994. During these first steps, several locations that might serve as a site for the large-scale airport were examined: Schönefeld-

---

[24] The members of the HIA team of the Institute of Public Health (*LÖGD*) North-Rhine Westphalia (NRW) conducted the interviews and the study in their capacity as participants in the effectiveness of HIA project. They performed their function as a working group reporting on the project from the German point of view but not in their function as *LÖGD* officials fulfilling tasks related directly to NRW.

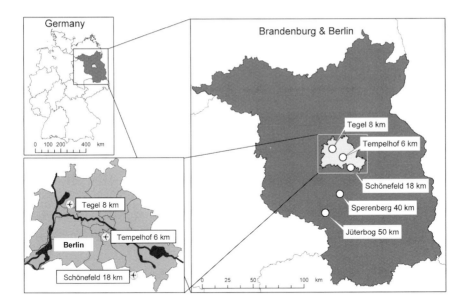

Figure CS11.1 *Overview of the most relevant airport sites close to Berlin*
Source: LÖGD, 2007

South, Jüterbog-East and Sperenberg (see Figure CS11.1). After different interests, risks and protection needs had been considered and balanced, there was a clear preference for the Sperenberg site.

The Schönefeld site was declared unsuitable due to its proximity to the densely populated south part of Berlin. Originally the projected airport was planned for an annual capacity of 60 million passengers including a non-stop 24-hour air service using four runways. An additional major evaluation criterion that backed the decision in favour of the more remote sites was the regional concept of decentralized concentration aimed at ensuring a balanced settlement structure in the State of Brandenburg and preventing a one-sided development of the area of Berlin (MIR, 2005).

This judgement of the situation changed fundamentally as a consequence of the state agreement on a joint regional planning policy for Greater Berlin-Brandenburg in 1995. In line with a change in policy direction, this development concentrated central functions in the cities of Berlin and Potsdam, complemented by further centres outside the planning area of Berlin. Thus the Schönefeld-South site became the most preferred option: located close to the city centre but not an inner-city site.

As early as 1996 as part of the consensual decision-making process (Gesellschafter BBF, 1996) the States of Berlin and Brandenburg and the Federal German Transport Ministry agreed on a concept focusing on the

Schönefeld airport extension. The modified plans included a reduced capacity of 30 million passengers per year and only two runways; a terminal building; traffic connections; and railway centre located between the two runways. On completion of the extended Schönefeld airport at the latest (schedule shifted from 2007 to 2011) the Berlin airports of Tempelhof and Tegel were to be closed. The extended airport is expected to have approximately 22 million passengers annually when air traffic begins in 2011.

The revised decision in favour of the Schönefeld site and subsequent application for construction approval started the procedure for the planning of a large-scale international airport at Berlin-Schönefeld. In 1999 Airport Berlin Schönefeld Ltd (partners: Federal Republic of Germany and the States of Berlin and Brandenburg) submitted the application for project approval, and this was published in February 2000. The assessment of future health effects in general followed the German planning standards for airport extension projects (*Planfeststellungsverfahren*), along with the planning procedures of airport extensions in Düsseldorf, Cologne/Bonn, Hahn or Frankfurt/Main.

Embedding HIA interventions in the BBI planning process

The process was not a predefined, foreseeable, well-organized HIA procedure. However, the stepwise progression of the planning procedure was accompanied by particular elements for assessing health effects that the LÖGD research team identified later as HIA elements. HIA procedures have been carried out since 2000, forecasting the future health situation of urban areas in neighbourhoods close to the extended airport. The assessment procedures focused on four major issues:

1 noise pollution and disturbance
2 pollution by noxious agents
3 accident risk
4 impacts on recreation.

The application for project approval was accompanied by several detailed expert opinions on these major health-relevant concerns.

Public participation started in spring 2001 as part of the draft proposal disclosure and the subsequent stakeholder hearing. Numerous institutions, associations and citizens made use of the opportunity to comment on the planning procedure, expressing their objections and views orally and in writing. Mostly they focused on the human health noise assessments included in the application for project approval. Opinions and contributions to the hearing procedures represented a broad range of views from national, state and regional levels, as well as from local actors and lobbyists. Those with concerns about the airport project were represented by organizations such as the Berlin Brandenburg Citizens' Association (BvBB), Association for Protecting the Interests of the Neighbouring Municipalities, and the German National Federation against Air Traffic Noise – using their own expertise and expert opinions. On the other side, the State Health Ministry of Brandenburg and the Health Authority of the Senate of Berlin commissioned separate studies on health-related concerns to support their statements with expert knowledge (Maschke & Hecht, 2000; Guski, 2000).

Further opinions on the examination of health concerns (in particular, human health noise assessments) submitted as part of the hearing process reflected the academic discussions on noise pollution research – a subject of great controversy in Germany.

Expected health-related impacts of the BBI project planning

The following is a short description of expected health-related impacts of the BBI project planning. This is presented as a synopsis of expert statements, expert opinions, objections and further sources such as contributions from the press, publications and the Internet. The explicit aims of the HIA process cannot be reported, as there is no official HIA procedure in Germany (Welteke & Machtolf, 2005; Fehr, Mekel & Welteke, 2004).

The BBI planning procedure was driven by clear intentions to meet the demands of human health protection to existing regulatory standards. While examining the HIA process for the Schönefeld site, it should be mentioned that one main political target was the closure of two city airports at Tegel and Tempelhof, with a resulting decrease in air traffic noise in their neighbourhoods.

Noise-induced health risks

While assessing the health consequences of air traffic noise, the primary expert opinion (Jansen, 2000a:M8) [25] defines several categories, scenarios, and settings related to the expected air traffic situation at the Schönefeld airport site. The primary expert opinion regarding health risks identifies a human threshold value of Leq3=85 dB(A) [26] for close-to-ear situations and for the deregulation of the vegetative nervous system a value of 19x99 dB(A) related to 19 single signals of air noise (daytime, outdoor) of 30 seconds extension each. The application for these noise-related health risks does not include any housing area.

---

[25] M8 and Mn are abbreviations relating to the series of primary expert opinions, which are part of the BBI project approval – see the references.

[26] This means that health impairments are expected if a noise intensity of 85 dB(A) is exceeded.

According to noise-related sleep disturbance symptoms, a maximum value Lmax of 6x75 dB(A) (night, outdoor) was set by the evidence-based findings (see footnote 26). These findings were the basis for determining an area of disturbance at night-time which gives information on the requirements for noise-protection measures. Another threshold value which marks the beginning of the relevant annoyance level is defined as Leq3 = 65 dB(A) (daytime; permanent noise level). If this value is exceeded, it increases significantly the percentage of people seriously affected. In addition to the area of disturbance at night-time, a nearly identical prevention area (permanent noise level of Leq3 = 62 dB(A)) was identified. By monitoring the data, a total of 111 exposure locations, 20 schools and 8 other noise sensitive institutions were identified in the disturbance area. For these sites, noise protection measures were recommended.

An additional expert opinion on noise pollution relates to aeroplane traffic at the airport and to other sources such as railway and highway traffic (Jansen, 2000b:M9). These effects are reported to occur at noise levels more than 10 dB(A) lower than those discussed for air traffic noise pollution. Therefore, the author of the findings states that this additional noise usually does not reach a level to affect health, that every source of noise leads to a specific and individual perception of noise and that a summarized category of overall noise is not sensible.

This background leads the author (Jansen, 2000a; Jansen, 2000b) to conclude that exorbitantly high levels of noise pollution affect only a couple of locations and institutions (for example, a school in Schönefeld itself – polluted by road traffic noise). These locations are said to require noise reduction measures with improved house insulation.

These primary findings in the planning approval received much criticism. There is doubt about the basic assumptions, calculating methods and those technical experts' opinions and prognoses (M1 prognosis and schedule of future air traffic; M3 expert opinion on physical noise extension; M4 noise pollution/environmental noise) which are the background of the noise-related M8 and M9 expert opinions. These arguments led to an expert dispute, initiated during the consultation procedure which culminated in the court hearing in Leipzig in February 2006. It reflects the German scientific community's long-term conflict about air noise which has accompanied several airport extension planning procedures and legal decisions in recent German history.

In addition, there have been arguments and discussions on scientific findings at expert hearings and panels preparing for Parliament's decision on a new air traffic noise act, which is to replace one from 1971. Additional input to this scientific discourse has been derived from the European decision on the EU Environmental Noise Directive (EU, 2002) and the national implementation of this legal framework. A brief selection of the central opposing arguments that have been put forward is given below.

The Ministry of Health Brandenburg (MASGF – in cooperation with the Ministry for Protection of the Environment Brandenburg) as an advocate of public (health) concerns commissioned two experts to prepare an extensive report (Maschke & Hecht, 2000). Their main conclusion is that the objectives of protection which are created and published in the M8 and M9 documents are regarded as inadequate according to updated prevention criteria of the German *Umweltbundesamt* – the Federal Environment Agency, Berlin (Ortscheid & Wende, 2000). The MASGF presented a series of preventive and threshold values which are documented in the extended version of the BBI case study (LÖGD, 2007).

If noise pollution levels exceed permanent noise values of 70 dB(A), resettlement measures for the affected residential population are recommended. With regard to the assessment of airport-induced ground-level noise, MASGF criticized the lack of a cumulative calculation of the overall burden of noise that usually contains the contribution of all sources of noise. Besides this, an assessment of ground-level noise pollution and its acoustic characteristics that uses only air-noise assessment criteria is said to produce an underestimation of the protection needs of the exposed population.

The Health Authority of the Senate of Berlin commissioned another report (Guski, 2000). This analyses a wide range of terms describing the technical area of "disturbance" and "annoyance" and concludes that social assessment criteria are much more reliable for planning procedure demands than parameters with a human health focus on air noise induced effects, which usually cannot prove causality to the suspected noxious sources. The report draws from questionnaire-based empirical research to state that the acoustic threshold value limiting non-tolerable annoyance by air traffic induced noise pollution should be at 59.5 dB(A) mean level in daytime.

The Federal Association Against Air Noise Pollution's statement raised several technical criticisms while assessing the expert opinions (M4) of the planning approval. Their critical focus related especially to the determination of incorrect small-sized noise pollution areas (Oeser & Beckers, 1999).

Defining objectives of noise protection

Basic approaches and recent findings have been the background of the above-mentioned critical responses and statements. In 2004 a decision of the Responsible Planning Administration Board (MSWV, 2004) ordered significant modification of the protection level in several points – deviating from the M8 and M9 recommendations. For example, the threshold value to prevent sleep disturbance is Lmax=55 dB(A) indoors which must not be exceeded more than six times per night. This is related to six outdoor noise events of Lmax=70 dB(A). If this threshold level is exceeded continuously, noise protection measures must be implemented (MSWV, 2004). Seven more categories, including a total of 24 single issues, are defined by setting concrete objectives for the adequate protection level.

In its decision of 16 March 2006, the Federal Administrative Court reacted to the numerous and serious concerns about expected health risks by imposing a ban on night flights between 24:00 and 05:00, a sentence following legislation which was applied in similar cases. Approval for the construction of the project was linked to conditions that refer to a review of the planning documentation and also involve further negotiations about additional hours of reduced air traffic (22:00–24:00 and 05:00–06:00).

Exposure to other agents

On this topic, the application for project approval drew from two different studies: the calculation and/or assessment of expected pollution levels (TÜV Rheinland/Berlin-Brandenburg, ARCADIS Trischler & Partner, 2000:M10) and their human-toxicological evaluation (Eikmann, 2000:M11). The following potential pollution sources were considered in detail and summarized in an overall conclusion:

• building site pollution (particularly from building site traffic)

• contribution to NO_2 pollution levels from central airport energy plants

• pollution from aircrafts and ground vehicles

• pollution from cars (airport-induced traffic).

All estimations were based on four model calculations with different scenarios developed for aircraft and ground-vehicle pollution. The pollutants and/or groups of pollutants considered were nitrogen oxides, airborne particles, soot and polycyclic aromatic hydrocarbons (PAH) with special consideration given to benzo(a)pyrene, benzene, toluene, ozone and carbon monoxide. Noxious smells and vibration levels were also taken into consideration.

The human-toxicological evaluation was based on model calculations and concluded that there is a danger of considerable exposure to harmful substances and odours on the airport site and in the direct vicinity (< 1 km) thus affecting parts of four neighbouring municipalities. However, this concerns mostly pollution from airport-induced vehicle traffic (NO_x, soot). Dust pollution levels during the construction phase were likely to be considerable in the area surrounding the airport – additional pollution for those parts of the municipalities already affected severely by noise pollution, and one that can hardly be minimized.

Critical comments indicate a lack of cumulative considerations for exposure in the primary expert opinion. Based on those assumptions, no elevated health risk was seen – not even for vulnerable people.

Accident risk

The flight-safety expert report (Fricke & Gronak, 2000: M21) dealt primarily with problems of safe airport operation as well as the required construction measures (flight-safety assessment). However, some items also related to health concerns: for example, as part of the assessments of accident risk on the ground; air levels of safety (LOS); the movement of wake vortices. With the help of model calculations, LOS were predicted internally (flight passengers and loading) and externally (local residents, employees working in the airport vicinity) for the extended airport, and also took into consideration endangering plants. The calculations resulted in an (annually) lethal accident risk of $< 10^{-5}$, which is comparable to similar-sized airports. The movement of wake vortices to populated areas was excluded due to the distances between runways and housing areas.

This expert opinion became the subject of much criticism because accident risk calculations had not included long-term injuries; LOS were used to draw conclusions about the timing of possible accidents; and there was no discussion of the fundamental uncertainties underlying such calculations (Wiesenthal, 2000).

Recreation areas

The impact on recreation was not considered in a separate primary expert opinion. The recreational areas affected by the airport extension are related to housing areas much larger than those areas analysed during the assessment of pollution effects. These recreational areas have been reliable resources for people looking for less (road traffic induced) noise and for relaxing from the stresses of everyday life. These sensible requirements have to be taken into account as a population effect which has to be balanced. The regional development plan for airport sites dating from 20 September 2005 has been working on these questions and presents an entire chapter on this issue (MIR, 2005).

Again, the assessment of health effects focuses on noise pollution. The main result is that the projected shifting of the runways to the south and an additional regulation on prohibiting direct crossings on BBI air routes would have positive effects on recreational areas situated in the north-east (e.g. Müggelsee). The effects on smaller green spaces (garden and park areas) were not analysed.

HIA process and context

Reviewing the HIA process

The entire process of assessing the health impact aspects of the BBI airport planning procedure was triggered by the transport policy decision to replace the three smaller Berlin airports with a single full-size airport.

The initial land-use planning procedure (ROV, completed 1994) was accompanied by a preliminary qualitative estimate of the health-related consequences of an international airport. The three alternative airport sites were assessed using population data for the surrounding housing areas. Apparently, there was no involvement of the health administration in this early stage; in German land-use planning, functional departments are usually consulted only if special issues arise.

After the *Konsensbeschluss* (political consensus decree) in 1996 (Gesellschafter BBF, 1996), the responsible project authority drew up the planning approval document for the extension of the existing Berlin-Schönefeld airport with the option for the future BBI airport. Although the scoping process heard advocates of public concerns, extended citizens' participation is not common in Germany at this stage of the process.

A special health assessment study (including long-term health effect analysis) was cancelled due to an alleged lack of methodological skills and specific legal requirements. In addition, the existing health monitoring baseline data of the Schönefeld area was seen as poor.[27] This had consequences for the performance of the ongoing HIA.

An HIA started in 1999 with a series of primary expert opinions commissioned by the responsible project bodies. The main focus was on statements concerning the health effects of noise pollution. These papers were presented as elements of the official planning approval that is compulsory in German planning

---

[27] A Health Impact Analysis going beyond the medical expertise on noise pollution and human-toxicological expertise is rejected by the responsible project bodies. In their opinion there was no legal basis for such an analysis. The possibility of such an analysis had been discussed and rejected during the scoping procedure, particularly since, according to statements by the responsible senate administrations and ministries, no previous data were available either. The examination of long-term impacts was to be assigned to the domain of basic research which had not to be done as part of an Environmental Impact Study (EIS). The material to be taken from the technical expertise was said to be sufficient for assessing the risks – particularly since parts of a Health Impact Analysis such as the analysis of the pollution situation do already exist and as the survey and assessment of the additional pollution were included in the expertise. The HIA steps required, according to Kobusch, Fehr & Serwe, were said to have been carried out as far as possible and as required. Moreover, a suitable methodology was said to be difficult to develop (Landesamt BVS Brandenburg, 2002; Kobusch, Fehr & Serwe, 1997).

procedures for major airport extension projects – and led to a series of long-term controversies.

Since the publication of the planning approval in February 2000, the commissioners of the planning process have had to balance the arguments of the conflicting parties and especially to deal with the allegation that the primary expert opinions led to an underestimation of health effects.[28]

The process of balancing the conflicts was dominated by different components with relevance to the later HIA outcome:

- Additional expert opinions and technical statements commissioned by advocates of public concerns and by actors of the housing population affected by the airport planning;

- Well-documented official hearing 2001/2002 of the 136 statements of the advocates of public concerns (31 days of hearing) and of the arguments of 130 000 objections from the affected population (59 days);

- Additional expert opinion on noise pollution exposure commissioned by the responsible planning authority in 2004 (Scheuch, 2004);

- The decision of the responsible planning authority: an 1171-page paper published in August 2004 including a modified set of threshold values.

There were significant differences in perceptions of the process. Members of the official institutions and the project management reported that the entire process, especially the participation and involvement of citizens' concerns, was managed according to the specific planning regulations; they pointed out that several processes of mediation were organized. Opponents of the airport extension reported their impression that they had had no real chance of influencing the results of the planning procedure. Notably, it was reported that the extensive hearings had no visible effect and there had been no mediation process.

In the last stage of the HIA-related process, the controversies were fought in the legal arena. First, there was an attempt to cancel the entire Schönefeld airport extension project by fighting the formal procedures used for the site selection (Supreme Court of Frankfurt/Oder). The March 2006 trial at the Federal Court of Leipzig was the final point of a legal controversy focusing, under HIA aspects, on the realization of a higher level of (noise) protection and prevention for the affected population.

---

[28] The extent of the conflict is visible when comparing the calculation of population numbers affected by the expected health consequences of air noise exposure. According to the primary expert opinion threshold values there is an affected population of approximately 40 000. The MASGF calculation identifies 80 000, another estimation commissioned by airport opponents assumes 120 000 persons will be affected.

HIA input and dynamics

Due to the extraordinary importance of the airport project, the entire planning process was accompanied by great attention from the public, political and economic arenas. There were several political decisions: (i) in favour of a single airport for Berlin (in connection with the foundation of a public company); (ii) reduction of the airport's original plans; (iii) 1996 decision in favour of the Schönefeld site. The third decision was made even though there was no doubt that many health conflicts would arise from planning an airport in a densely populated area. Several new plans on land-use regulation were commissioned in order to adjust the planning situation to modified political guidelines. Obviously, political attention accompanied the whole planning process. Following the Supreme Federal Court's March 2006 decision in favour of the realization of the Schönefeld airport extension plans, leading politicians commented that this was the most relevant decision for the east German economy.

The responsible project body commissioned several initiatives in order to facilitate the project, leading to positive health aspects for selected parts of the affected population (resettlement). In addition, there are social arguments in favour of the construction plans (Airport BBI as job engine, see LÖGD, 2007) – the medium term expectation of 40 000 additional jobs in the region.

Some interviewees reported that the main political influence seemed not to favour a thorough HIA procedure. The chosen primary expert opinion administrator on noise effects dominated the whole HIA-related process, which developed numerous antithetical statements to the criteria produced by the primary expert opinion.

Interviewees reported their impressions that the main influence of science and research in favour of HIA elements and input was organized and financed by actors from the affected population and several advocates of public concerns. Scientific input was implemented especially by expert opinions and hearings. A large amount of valuable scientific input was necessary to refute the values set by the primary expert opinion, while other fields of reasonable knowledge transfer became less important. Probably, more consistent legislation and regulation on the prevention of air noise pollution would have reduced the conflict. The HIA process elements were dominated by medical and scientific views with the exception of one expert opinion (Guski, 2000). Obviously, the broader WHO health definition and the inclusion of socioeconomic and social equity aspects played only a marginal role.

The input from legal practice on HIA matters has been of great influence. In particular, the verification that the planning procedure complied with existing objectives on noise pollution was seen as a useful intervention. Some interviewees argued the need for better tools to check this type of compliance in a more timely way in a preventive setting.

The public media's influence on HIA issues seemed to be reduced as a result of broad official political consensus in favour of the Schönefeld airport site. On the other hand, community pressure and dynamics have accompanied the entire HIA process since 2000. Interviewees stated that community influences were crucial for the realization of HIA core elements, e.g. there was a high level of public interest and control regarding the mode of action of those advocating public concerns. There seemed to be a great effort to organize expert opinions in favour of health protection issues. Considerable time and financial resources were activated in order to organize and facilitate participation, information transfer and the high level of legal dispute. Besides the demand in favour of establishing comprehensive HIA activities or elements, there was a strong community influence for making HIA performance more visible and popular. This was documented by numerous web pages reporting and commenting on relevant decisions and documents of HIA-related steps of the planning process.

From a broader perspective, the findings can be summarized as follows:

- There is a certain level of awareness of aspects of public health in German local settings but it is difficult to transform this into a solid political factor that is transferable into HIA routine procedures or local health plans.

- There are skills of analysis and assessment of expected (health) effects related to a concrete project or a project site planning – usually associated with EIA procedures. Decision-making processes that include health aspects at an early stage – e.g. while deciding on alternative sites – are presently an exception in Germany.

- Political influences that do not open their decision-making processes for participation and consideration of health aspects tend to create reasons for extended, conflicting, expensive and time-consuming planning procedures.

Conclusion

HIA dynamics

Due to the far-reaching implications of this planning project, especially for traffic policy and economics, assessment of the human-protection aspect was one important facet of the whole procedure. An additional HIA requested by some advocates of public interests was rejected explicitly. This rejection was repeated in the statement given after all the parties involved in the project had been heard.

During the advanced planning procedure, however, the particular topics of noise pollution and protection of the population affected played an extraordinary role in the decision-making process. Finally, the arguments of the advocates for public concerns and of the numerous opponents to the primary objectives of the planned project showed that only a modified plan could be realized at the Schönefeld site.

The planning authority and federal legal court had the task of balancing the conflicting arguments and mediating between the different interests. Depending on their personal points of view interviewees reported that mediation had been only more or less successful. Airport opponents unanimously saw the imposed air traffic restrictions during night hours as a partial success of their efforts. However, scepticism remained as it is felt that the dispute between the conflicting parties could be continued when interpreting and establishing the framework of the court's decision (e.g. related to the edge hours of the night traffic gap between 22:00 and 05:00).

This €2 billion project involving 15 years of planning procedures is a complex and extensive object for a case study. The huge area required for the construction of the airport and the extension of air and road traffic frequency in the region created some especially relevant HIA-related issues.

This HIA case study was facilitated by:

- enormous public attention;
- numerous expert opinions, especially on noise effects;
- good public information on the planning documents and expert opinions;
- positive and cooperative attitudes from actors involved;
- numerous HIA-related issues of relevance to national, regional and international settings and studies; and
- numerous findings expected from this case study with potential benefit and knowledge for other projects.

The Schönefeld project created a special conflicting situation that was complicated by shifting the former planning decision on the extension of the Sperenberg airport site which had had fewer negative implications for human health. Conflicting expert opinions on different noise reduction levels caused additional complications resulting in a breaking test for the entire project.

Dimensions of HIA effectiveness

Several problems and benefits affected the effectiveness of the HIA components and influencing factors accompanying the planning procedure and constituting the focus of this study.

- The lack of a systematic HIA procedure led to numerous expert opinions on health effects and probably contributed to an extended planning timetable (-).[29]

- Technical controversy about objectives of protection, threshold values (noise) and extension of prevention areas required extensive legal proceedings (-).

- Great efforts to meet technical standards of pollution measurement and assessment resulted in extensive data collection and an excellent initial position for an HIA (+).

- Great efforts to carry out the obligatory expert hearings and public participation led to an enormous number of well-documented statements and objections (+).

- Comprehensive pollution prognosis data and excellent initial position for HIA were not crucial for decision-making (-).

- Justified health demands of the population affected were finally (partly) successful in the federal court (+), but unsuccessful in the planning procedure itself (-).

The effectiveness of the HIA components is summarized below.

Health effectiveness: success in bringing important and justified health demands from the affected population (by legal proceedings) could be identified (+).

Community effectiveness: very strong in terms of the mobilization of citizens and community bodies in order to defend civil rights and health (by political, legal and technical defence) (+).

Equity effectiveness: has no final assessment, as the methodology available (interviews, analysing materials) failed to provide sufficient evidence for an evaluation (+/-).

Efficiency: These partially positive effects of health-related prognoses and evaluation procedures during project development and in the course of the lawsuit must be compared with the high amount of time-consuming financial, technical, scientific and emotional resources. The numerous expert opinions, potential underestimation of health impacts and the extensive legal proceedings caused by the lack of a regular and systematic HIA procedure displayed a high

---

[29] (+) and (-) are symbols for a positive or negative assessment related to HIA effectiveness.

grade of inefficiency leading to a time- and money-wasting procedure affecting all the actors involved.

The following strategies can be deduced for an increase in effectiveness and efficiency (lessons to be learned in Germany):

1 Stronger orientation of German planning procedures towards international good-practice models, e.g. according to integrated HIA skills and elements.
2 Strengthen proactive HIA routines.
3 Stronger focus on management and mediation aspects in order to induce early and appropriate consideration and communication of health aspects.
4 Better technical clarification and legal determination of protection target levels before a project starts (also addresses to the German legislative bodies).
5 Pay more attention to preventive techniques (like HIA) and conflict resolution skills in order to manage and negotiate controversies in the context of planning procedures rather than afterwards in extensive legal proceedings.

These findings are in line with the recommendations for the future development of a German HIA, which resulted from an international HIA workshop held in November 2001 in Berlin (Welteke & Fehr, 2002). The BBI case study presented some insights into a planning process that was characterized by intense technical controversy, and by a time- and resource- consuming procedure that adapted HIA elements only in a predominantly reactive way.

Health aspects were seen to be important in the planning procedure and in the ensuing lawsuits. This supports the argument that similar planning projects should be provided with earlier, well-defined, preventive, proactive and better-organized HIA components. In addition, the role of the legislation must be reflected in such tools as a stronger legal basis is necessary to define and realize adequate and compulsory protection objectives.

REFERENCES

Eikmann T (2000). *Gutachten über die Auswirkungen der flughafenbedingten Schadstoffimmissionen (Humantoxikologisches Gutachten)*. Abschnitt **M11** des Antrags auf Planfeststellung zum Ausbau Flughafen Schönefeld. Wetzlar, Gesellschaft für Umwelttoxikologie und Krankenhaushygiene mbH.

EU (2002). Directive 2002/49/EC of the European Parliament and the Council of 25 June 2002 relating to the assessment and management of environmental noise. *Official Journal of the European Communities*, L189:12–25.

Fehr R, Mekel O, Welteke R (2004). HIA: the German perspective. In: Kemm J, Parry J, Palmer S, eds. *Health impact assessment*. Oxford & New York, Oxford University Press:253–264.

Fricke M, Gronak N (2000). *Flugsicherheitsgutachten*. Abschnitt **M21** des Antrags auf Planfeststellung zum Ausbau Flughafen Schönefeld. Berlin, Gesellschaft für Luftverkehrsforschung bR.

Gesellschafter BBF (1996). *Konsensbeschluss vom 28.05.1996.* Berlin, Gesellschafter der Berlin-Brandenburg Flughafen Holding GmbH (http://www.buergerbewegung.de/konsens.htm, accessed 4 April 2006).

Guski R (2000). *Stellungnahme zu den medizinischen Gutachten M8 und M9 bezüglich des Ausbaus des Flughafens Schönefeld vom 21.06.2000.* Bochum, Auftrag der Berliner Senatsverwaltung für Arbeit, Soziales und Frauen.

Jansen G (2000a). *Medizinisches Gutachten über die Auswirkungen des Fluglärms auf die Bevölkerung in der Umgebung des Flughafens Schönefeld.* Abschnitt **M8** des Antrags auf Planfeststellung zum Ausbau Flughafen Schönefeld, o. O.

Jansen G (2000b). *Medizinisches Gutachten über die Auswirkungen der flughafenbedingten Geräusche auf die Bevölkerung.* Abschnitt **M9** des Antrags auf Planfeststellung zum Ausbau Flughafen Schönefeld, o. O.

Kobusch AB, Fehr R, Serwe HJ, eds (1997). *Gesundheitsverträglichkeitsprüfung.* Baden-Baden, Grundlagen, Konzepte, Praxiserfahrungen Hrsg.

Landesamt BVS Brandenburg (2002). *Stellungnahme – Ergebnis des Anhörungsverfahrens Ausbau Flughafen Berlin-Schönefeld vom 14.06.2002.* Potsdam, Landesamt für Bauen, Verkehr und Straßenwesen Brandenburg.

LÖGD (2007). *bbi case study – Annexes.* Bielefeld, LÖGD NRW (http://www.loegd.nrw.de/bbicase, accessed 21 March 2007).

Maschke C, Hecht K (2000). *Gutachterliche Stellungnahme zu den lärmmedizinischen Gutachten M8 und M9 "Ausbau Flughafen Schönefeld" vom 09.06.2000.* Berlin, Auftrag des Ministeriums für Arbeit, Soziales, Gesundheit und Frauen des Landes Brandenburg.

MIR (2005). *Landesentwicklungsplan Flughafenstandortentwicklung (LEP FS) ergänzendes Verfahren.* (Entwurf in der Fassung vom 20 September 2005.) Potsdam, Ministerium für Infrastruktur und Raumordnung des Landes Brandenburg, Senatsverwaltung für Stadtentwicklung Berlin.

MSWV (2004). *Planfeststellungsbeschluss Ausbau Verkehrsflughafen Berlin-Schönefeld 44/1-6441/1/101 vom 13.08.2004.* Potsdam, Ministerium für Stadtentwicklung, Wohnen und Verkehr des Landes Brandenburg.

Oeser K, Beckers HJ (1999). *Fluglärm 2000. 40 Jahre Fluglärmbekämpfung – Forderungen und Ausblick.* Düsseldorf, Bundesvereinigung gegen Fluglärm, Springer VDI.

Ortscheid J, Wende H (2000). *Fluglärmwirkungen.* Berlin, Umweltbundesamt.

Scheuch K (2004). *Lärmmedizinische Stellungnahme im Rahmen des Planfeststellungsverfahrens für den Ausbau des Verkehrsflughafens Berlin-Schönefeld vom 05.07.2004.* Bannewitz, Auftrag des Ministeriums für Stadtentwicklung, Wohnen und Verkehr des Landes Brandenburg.

TÜV Rheinland/Berlin-Brandenburg, ARCADIS Trischler & Partner (2000). *Gutachten über Schadstoffimmissionen.* Abschnitt **M10** des Antrags auf Planfeststellung zum Ausbau Flughafen Schönefeld. Köln, TÜV Rheinland/Berlin-Brandenburg, ARCADIS Trischler & Partner.

Welteke R, Fehr R, eds (2002). *Workshop Gesundheitsverträglichkeitsprüfung Health Impact Assessment. Im Rahmen des Aktionsprogrammembers Umwelt und Gesundheit (APUG).* Berlin, 19 und 20 Nov 2001. Bielefeld, Tagungsband.

Welteke R, Machtolf M (2005). Gesundheitsverträglichkeit von Projekten und Planungen. In: Fehr R, Neus H, Heudorf U, eds. *Gesundheit und Umwelt. Ökologische Prävention und Gesundheitsförderung.* Bern, Verlag Hans Huber:210–219.

Wiesenthal H (2000). *Risikowissenschaftliche Bewertung des Flugsicherheitsgutachtens für den Ausbau des Flughafens Schönefeld* **(M21)**. Berlin.

Case study 12

"Buzz" around electromagnetic fields: a lengthy environmental HIA in Poland

Anicenta Bubak[30] and Ewa Nowak

Introduction

Community protests have the potential to lengthen and impact on decision-making processes regarding health impact assessment (HIA). This case study shows that all community protests should be taken into account, even if this requires additional and long-term procedures. In this case, the environmental health impact assessment (EHIA) was incorporated adequately into the decision-making process.

The case study concerns a proposed mobile phone base station sited on a school building. The case of Bartoszyce was selected from the EHIA cases in Poland as it has been used as a precedent and is an example of the practice of good health procedures for the whole country.

The main potential health hazard was electromagnetic fields (EMF). The impact on human health due to EMF from mobile masts raises fears and emotions in the public at large. The use of mobile telephones and the number of transmitters have increased considerably in recent years. Over the period of the study, there were substantial community complaints about the siting of mobile-phone antennae in Poland (Table CS12.1).

---

[30] Expert from National Reference Centre on Environmental Health Impact Assessment – opinion concerning EHIA procedure (2005).

Table CS12.1 *Number of community complaints during the case study period*

Year	No of cases
2004	200
2005	410
2006 (two months)	100

Source: Data from interview with administrator representing the Minister of the Environment.

This chapter proceeds as follows: the first section addresses the background of the Bartoszyce case; the second discusses the aims of the EHIA, and its effectiveness from three perspectives: health, equity and community; the third gives more detail on the EHIA process and context. It concludes by examining positive and negative factors for the effectiveness of the EHIA.

Profiling the EHIA

This case study concerns a prospective local EHIA connected with the telecommunication sector in a county town in Warmia and Mazury Voivodeship in north-east Poland, near the border with Kaliningrad Province (Russia). Bartoszyce covers an area of 11 km² and is an important region for tourism and the transport of goods. It has 28 000 inhabitants: 14 700 female and 13 300 male (27% below working age). In the town of Bartoszyce, a mobile phone base station antenna was planned to be situated on the school building which is surrounded by apartment buildings.

The potential health hazards centred on the EMF emitted from the mobile antenna and noise caused by its installation. EMF induce thermal and non-thermal effects in living organisms. EMF exposures below the limits recommended in the standards do not appear to have any known consequence on human health. The Ordinance of the Ministry of Environment regulates the maximum level of EMF in the environment and related monitoring (Dziennik Ustaw, 2003). It was necessary to estimate the potential EMF hazards for human health in such a location before deciding whether to erect the mobile phone antenna. The Mayor carried out the EHIA between 2004 and 2006.

In Poland, the legal basis for HIA is provided in the Environmental Protection Law (Dziennik Ustaw, 2001). The State Sanitary Inspection Act complements this law and describes the rules of health protection and the HIA report evaluation (Dziennik Ustaw, 1985). A third act – the Code of Administrative Procedure – determines the administrative process (Dziennik Ustaw, 2000).

HIA is a part of both social impact assessment (SIA) and environmental impact assessment (EIA). According to article 47, point 1a of the Environmental Protection Law (Dziennik Ustaw, 2001):

In the environmental impact assessment procedure, the following shall be identified, analysed and assessed: the direct and indirect effects of a given project on the environment, *human health and the quality of human life,* the interaction between environmental, health and other factors, the possible ways of preventing, reducing adverse impacts on the environment and health, and the monitoring, as required.

This act ensures access to environmental information (part IV, articles 19–24) and public participation (part V, articles 31–39). The public investments for which the EHIA report is obliged to are based on screening criteria listed in the Ordinance of the Council of Ministries (Dziennik Ustaw, 2002).

This case study is based on interviews with four stakeholders who took part in the decision-making process, and documents related to the preparation of the decision and EHIA. These include reports and correspondence from residents and local, regional and state-level institutions that took part in the procedure.

The first interviewee was an executive officer responsible for decisions at the local governmental level, representing the Mayor. The second was a key actor responsible for health issues, who participated in scoping and evaluating the EHIA report, representing the Voivodeship Sanitary Inspectorate (VSI). The other two interviewees were senior administrators from institutions of higher level in the procedure. One was the administrator responsible for environmental and health issues, a WHO expert in electromagnetic fields who represented the Ministry of the Environment (MoE). The other interviewee was an authority in health issues concerning EMF (mainly mobile phone antennae) from the Chief Sanitary Inspectorate (CSI).

Aims of the EHIA

The main aim of the EHIA was to predict, assess and minimize potential negative effects on human health caused by EMF emitted from the planned antenna at the school building. The EHIA resulted in approval of the decision to locate the mobile phone antenna on the school building, following the positive appraisals conducted by the Voivodeship and the CSI. A decision was made despite community protests because it was recognized that this location, its distance from surrounding buildings and the EMF intensity would have no harmful effects on human health.

The decision about the conditions of the antenna's location was first taken in 2005, because of a lack of harmful effects on human health in a probable area for the maximum level of EMF (established or fixed by the maximum power of the antenna). The EHIA process was extended due to community protests and appeals were involved in this process and the decision to allow the erection of the mobile phone antenna was taken in 2006.

Dimensions of effectiveness

Health effectiveness

The health impact was a central theme in the assessment. Based on the opinion of the four interviewees, there was general health effectiveness. The health aspect addressed by the EHIA was acknowledged adequately in the decision-making process but did not modify the decision as no negligible health effects were reported. Three interviewees (representatives of the Mayor, VSI and MoE respectively) stated: " … the report acknowledges, health impacts are negligible or rather positive".

In the EHIA report, the main hazards connected with the mobile antenna were the EMF and noise. The probable area of the maximum EMF level in the environment was fixed by the maximum power usage of the antenna. EMF levels were lower than those determined by Polish and European standards. The levels of EMF could be higher than environmental standards only in the area closest to the antenna (e.g. where maintenance duties are carried out) therefore methods to protect against harmful effects were proposed for occupational exposure only. The recommendations for those employed on maintenance, control and breakdowns of the installation included limiting EMF exposure time and regular medical examinations. Additionally, the VSI determined conditions concerning the height of the mast bearing in mind the protection of children, although there is a lack of medical evidence showing different responses to EMF for various population groups.

One interviewee (responsible for health issues at regional level) suggested that although the EHIA did not affect the decision, it raised awareness among policy-makers. National experts in EHIA (EHIA, biology, biophysics, EMF and law specialists; environmental/occupational physicians) were asked for their opinions on the local community's fears concerning the human health impacts of mobile antennae and EMF. These experts evaluated the materials delivered by the local community as irrational and non-scientific, and gave additional opinions about EMF, the EHIA report and the attached documents.

Based on this additional expertise, this EHIA is used regionally and nationally as a precedent for other cases where EMF from mobile phone antennae are likely to cause a buzz.

Equity effectiveness

The interviewees perceived equity from the perspective of "taking age and special groups into consideration" and "equity of access to environmental and health information, public participation in the decision-making process". All interviews pointed to direct effectiveness because the pending decision was postponed until additional expertise could respond to the fears of affected residents. The protestors reacted by utilizing their rights of access to justice in environmental matters (Dziennik Ustaw, 2000).

All interviewees considered that equity standards were taken into consideration in this procedure. Local residents lodged complaints against the antenna at regional and state levels with environmental and health institutions.

The MoE administrator gave a further comment concerning equity: "According to WHO guidelines, there is no special age or vulnerable groups in cases of EMF hazards".

Community effectiveness

Public participation is an instrument applied by community organizations and nongovernmental organizations (NGOs) and respected by different levels of the Polish government. Community effectiveness is understood as a transparent EHIA process; interviewees perceived this case to have general community effectiveness. The Mayor directly and indirectly informed the community about the planned antenna, and there was contact with the community during the procedure.

According to the interviewees, the community's stance did not affect the decision as it was dismissed as groundless or ambiguous. Community opinion did not produce a change and the decision was contrary to their expectations. This EHIA required special scientific opinion to help place rational arguments above the fears of the community. National experts of the EHIA judged the community stance to be based on irrational and non-scientific arguments.

Such community doubts were in line with similar cases connected with mobile antennae in Poland and other countries, not only in Europe. One interviewee, the MoE administrator, cited evidence that the community was informed adequately about health consequences, suggesting that Polish standards (EMF in environment) are more protective than the EU and the decision was transparently supported by this information.

Other dimensions of effectiveness

The EHIA was not cost-effective – it was expensive and the additional legal

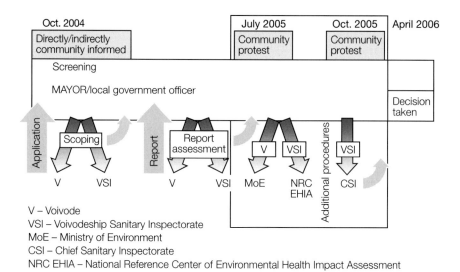

Figure CS12.1 *Main phases of the Bartoszyce mobile phone antenna EHIA procedure*

and scientific opinions increased the costs. Yet it shows procedural effectiveness despite a long and complicated procedure caused by community protest. It gives a precedent for good health procedural practices for related cases in Poland and, in this context, was cost-effective for the next EHIA in this field. The EHIA also demonstrated effectiveness for cooperation between the health services and scientists concerning the evaluation and evidence-based information about EMF health hazards.

Effectiveness is also linked to the way in which officials engage in the procedural work, their attitudes and liability. In this case, they engaged sincerely in their duties and scientific capacities of the research were readily available.

Process, input and context of EHIA

Process

The EHIA process started according to the usual procedure (Figure CS12.1). The investor – the mobile phone operator – applied for permission to the Mayor of Bartoszyce in October 2004. The local government officer responsible for land use, a representative of the Mayor, informed the community directly and indirectly about the planned antenna via the media and letters (to neighbours and interested parties). Simultaneously, he conducted a screening and made the decision that the case should be run under the EHIA procedure.

The officer asked for input from Warmian and Mazurian Voivode (V) on the environmental impact scope and VSI for the health impact scope. In the time required by law, both institutions sent their opinions concerning the scope of the report to the Mayor. These were the basis for the report prepared by the consultant hired by the investor. The report defined the main hazards associated with EMF and noise emitted from mobile antenna. The probable area of the maximum level of EMF in the environment was established using the maximum power of the antenna. The report stated that this location would produce no harmful effects on human life – any effects would relate to occupational exposure only; and listed proposals for avoiding these harmful effects. The investor submitted the report to the Mayor. This was released to the public and then appraised by *V* (environmental impact) and VSI (health impact) in EHIA reports that were delivered to the Mayor's office.

VSI produced a positive EHIA report. The assessment proposed restrictions on future use of land with potential EMF in Bartoszyce and for new buildings near the antenna. In such cases, the power of the antenna has to be reduced or stopped to make the area free of EMF.

In July 2005 local community representatives protested against the mobile phone antenna because they believed that EMF might have harmful effects on the environment and human health. This community stance triggered additional procedures. The community sent their comments on *V*'s positive EHIA report to the Ministry of Environment, which kept in force the assessment. VSI asked the National References Centre of Environmental Health Impact Assessment (NRCEHIA) for additional opinions about their EHIA report and attached materials. NRCEHIA evaluated materials delivered by the protesting community as irrational and non-scientific.

Simultaneously, the community requested the cancellation of VSI's assessment concerning EMF and noise-related health effects. The CSI upheld the assessment. Finally, the Mayor took the decision and accepted the planned mobile phone siting.

Input and context

The driving force behind the EHIA came from legal and administrative levels, the local government officer responsible for the decision-making process and community dynamics. VSI provided direction and leadership throughout the procedure; specifically, the Preventive Sanitary Department with Radiology.

The additional procedures involved three independent steering groups:

1 NRCEHIA group prepared assessment with concern for health determinants, based on medical data on diseases caused by EMF.

2 Environmental and EMF experts (WHO) working in the MoE.
3 Environmental, radiological and health experts and a lawyer from the CSI in the Ministry of Health.

This additional procedure was triggered by community fears that had been multiplied by the activity of the NGO, the Association against Electrohazards. The investor, local government and State Sanitary Inspectorate budgets covered the costs. There were no political or other interventions in favour or against the EHIA, although it took place during parliamentary and presidential elections.

Conclusion

Environmental and health authorities in Poland discussed the health definition taken into account by EHIA. New qualitative and quantitative methodologies of risk assessment were developed. Practices in public participation and access to information about plans, programmes and projects relating to the environment and health still need to be improved in Poland. The community is using the rights assured by law, but is not always able to appraise the real health hazards and sometimes is confused by information from dubious sources. In this case, one interviewee played the role of official mediator and tried to explain the residents' arguments concerning mobile phone antennae and EMF hazards. The residents did not accept mediator's arguments, and represented the standpoint of the NGO, the Association against Electrohazards. Although it is illegal in Poland a rising number of people disseminate counterfeit information which causes panic in the community. This is popularized via web pages registered on foreign servers.

The interviewees expressed the necessity for basic ecological and health education, which should be spread throughout all social groups in the community. The mass media could inform the general public about environmental and health hazards, especially radiation and EMF. The educational system should involve environmental and health authorities. All these actions might help to decrease community protests caused by strong, but often groundless, fears.

The National Ecological Policy's aims for EMF are to create a monitoring system and a database about environmental levels of EMF, and to develop administrative procedures ensuring safe locations for EMF sources and a reference laboratory on EMF measurement.

This is not just a problem for Poland, as noted by WHO (WHO, 2006):

> Because disparities in EMF standards around the world have caused increasing public anxiety about EMF exposures from the introduction of new technologies, WHO commenced a process

of harmonization of EMF standards worldwide. With 54 participating countries and 8 international organizations involved in the EMF Project, it provides a unique opportunity to bring countries together to develop a framework for harmonization of EMF standards and to encourage the development of exposure limits and other control measures that provide the same level of health protection to all people.

REFERENCES

Dziennik Ustaw (1985). Law on State Sanitary Inspection (No. 12, item 49 with amendment).

Dziennik Ustaw (2000). Law on Code of Administrative Procedure (No. 98, item 1071 with amendment).

Dziennik Ustaw (2001). Law on Environmental Protection (No. 62, item 627 with amendment).

Dziennik Ustaw (2002). Ordinance of the Council of Ministries on the screening criteria of public investments for preparing Environmental Impact Assessment reports (No. 179, item 1490).

Dziennik Ustaw (2003). Ordinance of the Ministry of Environment concerning the maximum level of electromagnetic fields in the environment and the way of monitoring (No. 192, item 1883).

WHO (2006) [web site]. Electromagnetic fields, standards and guidelines (EMF Project). Geneva, World Health Organization (http://www.who.int/peh-emf/standards/en/, accessed 1 June 2006).

Part V
The Effectiveness of Elements of Health Impact Assessment: Case Studies

Case study 13

Pushing the agenda among decision-makers: an international assessment of transport-related health effects in six countries

Martin Sprenger and Ursula Püringer

Introduction

In Austria, Health Impact Assessment (HIA) is usually translated as *Gesundheitsverträglichkeitsprüfung* (GVP). This is an imitation of the more common and official term *Umweltverträglichkeitsprüfung* (UVP), which is the widely accepted official translation of EIA. In contrast to UVP there is no legal basis for a GVP; many stakeholders would claim that most UVPs integrate an assessment of health impacts (Arbter, 2004; BGBl, 2002). However, the literal translation is inadequate, as GVP and HIA use different methods and concepts, and involve different actors. Assessments of acceptability from a health perspective (so called GVPs) often focus on single diseases, work with a narrow definition of health, and are often expert-based, mono-disciplinary medical assessments limited to the mere identification of environmental risks.

The Austrian team was responsible for the overall project coordination of their case study which describes a transnational project (Austria, France, Malta, the Netherlands, Sweden and Switzerland) that started in 2003. The project on transport-related health effects with a particular focus on children is one of the first outcomes of the Transport, Health and Environment (THE) Pan-European Programme (PEP). The aims of the project were (i) to provide an integrated assessment on the state of the art on transport-related health impacts, costs and benefits and (ii) to make a set of evidence-based recommendations on political implementation strategies with particular attention to the needs of children.

As THE PEP states:

> Efficient transport systems are essential for the growth of our economies and the mobility of our people. However, the current trends in transport development challenge sustainable development, resulting in large detrimental health and environmental impacts that to a disproportionate extent affect the most vulnerable and particularly children (Bundesministerium für Land- und Forstwirtschaft Umwelt- und Wasserwirtschaft (BMLFUW), 2004).

The project reviewed the scientific literature on the major transport-related health effects on children (air pollution, noise, physical activity, psychological aspects, road injuries, climate change). It also facilitated a series of four two-day workshops with the participation of experts and stakeholders on health, transport, environment, economy and children's affairs; scientists, NGO and government representatives from the Organisation for Economic Co-operation and Development (OECD), United Nations Economic Commission for Europe (UNECE), United Nations Environment Programme (UNEP), WHO and others. An online comprehensive brochure covers the main outcomes, conclusions and recommendations (Bundesministerium für Land- und Forstwirtschaft Umwelt- und Wasserwirtschaft (BMLFUW), 2004). The results were also presented at the fourth WHO Ministerial Conference on Environment and Health, the Future for our Children, held in Budapest on 23–25 June 2004.

The selected case study is interesting for the following reasons. First, the programme was initiated by a single person from the Austrian Federal Ministry of Agriculture, Forestry, Environment and Water. Second, its clear aims were to influence politicians and other decision-makers at the fourth WHO Ministerial Conference on Environment and Health and to push and influence WHO's Children's Environment and Health Action Plan for Europe (CEHAPE). However, this is a debatable case study as it does not judge the potential population health effects of a policy, programme or project and therefore is not a classic HIA according to the definition in the Gothenburg consensus paper (European Centre for Health Policy, 1999). For this reason the term assessment is used rather than HIA throughout the text.

This chapter provides the reader with the what, where and when of the assessment and the context of the country in which it took place. We interviewed three experts involved in the project to obtain more insight into its process and outcomes (effectiveness). This was an international project which aimed to assess present and future European transport development in terms of its potential effects on the health of the affected European population (primarily children), and to integrate environmental and health dimensions into future European transport policies.

Context of the assessment

In Austria, a variety of procedures, methods and tools are used for judging a policy, programme or project's potential effects on the health of individuals, as well as the wider population. At present, there is no database where all these assessments are collected systematically.

Motorized road transport is increasing rapidly in the European region; further rises are anticipated with the economic development in eastern Europe. Austria is affected extensively by transit and transport policies due to its geographical location, so most assessments (environmental impact assessment (EIA), strategic environmental impact assessment (SEIA), etc.) are aimed at this sector. Austria has undertaken or participated in several studies on the health impact of traffic, especially overall air pollution since 1999, and has utilized some creative approaches, e.g. measuring health costs per kilometre of road built. However, the lack of consistent methods to assess the overall health impacts of transport policies has led to a conglomeration of different approaches, ranging from narrow mono-disciplinary expert opinions to comprehensive interdisciplinary assessments and recommendations. This applies to local, regional and national levels.

As mentioned above, during the interviews it became clear that the driving force behind this assessment was an individual from the Austrian Federal Ministry of Agriculture, Forestry, Environment and Water. Personal contacts from a previous project (the Tri-national European project of Austria, France and Switzerland for WHO's London Conference in 1999) have been very important to the realization of this transnational project and obtaining financial support from the national authorities: UNECE, OECD and WHO. Interestingly the EU provided no financial support; interviewees explained this as a denial of WHO. There have been great differences in the financial support from national authorities, e.g. Switzerland provided many more resources than France; other project partners provided Malta with financial support in order to participate in and facilitate the final workshop.

No explicit definition of HIA has been used in this particular case study. The work was based on an intersectoral and interdisciplinary approach. After the assessment had been commissioned and a steering group established, every country worked independently to look at special transport-related health effects. The ability to work as a team was enhanced by professional project management, with the allocation of roles, tasks, resources, timetables, meetings and deadlines.

Interviewees were clear that an assessment of transport-related health effects can be effective only when transport is considered as an international issue, and tries directly to influence European transport policy. The project brought together not only experts, scientists and other stakeholders on health, transport, environment, economy and children's affairs from NGOs and government institutions in six different countries, but also involved international organizations such as the OECD, UNECE, UNEP and WHO.

The very tight time frame presented organizational constraints and programme limitations. From the start in 2003 the project team had a clear end-point for presenting the results: the WHO Ministerial Conference in Budapest 23–25 June 2004. One interviewee noted that some effects of transport, such as the contamination of soil and water, were not included because of these time constraints.

The assessment examined transport as an international issue and therefore used a different approach for screening, scoping, appraising and reporting. For example, the project did not consider regional distinctions and there was no community involvement.

Below we describe the process and the outcome (effectiveness) of this assessment of present and future European transport development.

Aim of the assessment and dimensions of effectiveness

The aim of producing an integrated assessment of transport-related health effects was achieved through the following endeavours:

- focusing on children;

- highlighting potential costs and benefits;

- looking at methodological aspects, e.g. unifying the calculation of health-related external costs;

- giving policy directions to address transport-related health effects on children;

- selecting pertinent health effects on children to estimate the quantitative relationships between exposure and health effects (exposure response function);

- estimating accurately the fraction of exposure from transport;

- measuring and expressing in monetary terms the effects of physical, mental and social health and well-being to achieve comparability.

The main determinants were linked to the physical environment (air pollution, climate change, road traffic injuries, noise), but also the assessment looked at lifestyles (physical activity). Although psychological and social determinants were not considered in great detail the assessment considered the psychological and social effects of other determinants.

Each participating country appraised transportation developments using the following criteria, with a focus on health effects:

Austria – psychological and social effects.

France – air pollution (e.g. exacerbation of asthma, chronic respiratory symptoms, allergic symptoms, increased prevalence of atopic sensations, reductions in lung function).

Malta – climate change and road traffic injuries.

The Netherlands – noise (e.g. sleep disturbance, effects on children's learning, cognition, motivation and annoyance).

Sweden – economic evaluation.

Switzerland – physical activity (obesity, positive effects on psychological and physical well-being).

According to one interviewee, several studies have tried to prove the direct health effects of transport-related noise and pollution on children, but the dose-effect relation seems to be somewhat arbitrary and can only be estimated. As there had been no systematic literature research on psychosocial effects, the Austrian project team carried out a comprehensive analysis of the literature on the psychosocial effects of traffic noise, stressors, accidents and their consequences (e.g. post-traumatic stress disorders (PTSD)) for children and their carers.

The assessment was effective in its aim to undertake an integrated assessment of transport-related health effects on children and present the findings at the WHO conference. The six countries presented an extensive assessment, thereby putting the focus on health effects on children and making the issue more relevant to politicians.

Interviewees noted that a strong economic focus – looking at economic costs and making them transparent – was essential in order to push the agenda among politicians. Economic arguments are crucial for health-related issues to pass international bodies and parliaments (e.g. EU Commission, EU Parliament). The assessment was also successful in using new approaches in the assessment of transport-related health effects (e.g. risk value, willingness to pay, sensitivity analyses, unification of the calculation of health-related external costs). One interviewee identified a limitation – there were many interesting single outcomes of the project, but no comprehensive overview.

One interviewee stated that intelligent transport and mobility management is taking place more often in Austria. Action papers have been launched, CO_2 emissions reduced, and measures to reduce transport-related health effects (noise, air pollution, traffic-related injuries) have been financed and implemented. Health effects are incorporated more often in big projects (such as those addressing transport, urban planning). One interviewee said that the assessment changed transport policies in Austria and argued that the same could be true for other countries.

The Austrian Ministry of Women and Health published a brochure on Healthy Environment for Our Children (Bundesministerium für Land- und Forstwirtschaft Umwelt- und Wasserwirtschaft (BMLFUW), 2005) containing recommendations such as bicycle lanes to increase safety and physical activity. Austrian politicians are exploring ways to take account of the full cost, including externalities, of new policies, e.g. introducing higher road charges to recover the cost of transport investment.

One important outcome at European level was a set of key messages and policy directions addressing different aspects of transport-related effects on environment and health, which were included in CEHAPE.

Interviewees felt some scepticism about the assessment's effectiveness in boosting transport-related health effects on the agendas of UNECE, OECD, large EU freight companies, economic departments, and so on. It was also felt to be ineffective at informing the public through easy to understand communication tools (social marketing). This is a great pity as the final report is well written and should be distributed more widely.

While the assessment was not directly effective with regard to health, it raised awareness among policy-makers and may have changed some policies. The final report has been written in eight languages and gives clear recommendations in the form of key messages and policy directions. Some of these recommendations are already in place in some countries, e.g. incentives for zero or ultra-low emission vehicles (noise, pollution).

Equity was not a main issue in this assessment. This reflects a large gap in the assessment of transport-related health effects, as these are higher in vulnerable groups (e.g. low-income, children, migrants) given that they are more likely to work and live close to railways, roads, etc. Social equity is an important issue that has not been considered in the economic evaluation of transport-related health effects. Some project partners wanted to include questions of equity on the agenda, but failed to do so. It was not possible to obtain more detailed information on the underlying reasons.

The assessment was not directly effective on community issues, as no community was involved. The assessment remains expert and scientifically based. Selective groups of potentially affected populations (children) were given questionnaires or participated in interviews for psychology students' Master's theses. It cannot be judged whether this sample is representative. However, the assessment may have been indirectly effective: for example, community activists in Austria are using the results and recommendations to lobby against transit and transport policies.

The process of the assessment

The assessment was planned with a clear aim (to assess transport-related health effects on children) and a clear end-point (the WHO conference).

After the initial work of the Austrian project team, all project partners worked together on screening. Each project country carried out independent scoping and appraisal of special transport-related health effects. The project team used standard two- to three-day workshops, organized by each country, to discuss the different health effects, scoping and appraisal methods and to help each project partner to finalize their work. This approach was cost-effective and allowed the project team to work intensively and efficiently. The workshops brought together experts, scientists and other stakeholders on health, transport, environment, economy and children's affairs from NGOs and government institutions and representatives from international organizations such as the OECD, UNECE, UNEP and WHO.

Reporting and evaluation have been done together, although the project management team in Austria condensed the comprehensive paperwork (input-reports) into understandable and readable reports and presentations for politicians and the public (output-reports).

The company responsible for overall project coordination has a long tradition of traffic planning and economic evaluation of transport (e.g. road pricing) and has professional links with national and international organizations in this field. However, this expertise meant that the assessment developed a strong economic focus on the costs and benefits of transport-related health effects on children.

While there was no community participation, communities and organizations used reports and arguments (using key messages) to advocate their interests. Many people were involved. The impressive number of well-known people from public health, health and environment research, health policy and science was an effective tool for advocating the issue at national and international levels.

The final report was achieved as a team effort. It was presented at the fourth WHO Ministerial Conference on Environment and Health – The Future for our Children in Budapest, 23–25 June 2004. It received much attention and a positive reception. Each country has produced national reports; delivered national presentations, published in the national media; and taken part in press conferences, talk shows and related media outlets. Web pages have been established to make the full text reports available for download.

Conclusion

As noted previously, the assessment would not have taken place without the engagement of a single individual at the Ministry of Agriculture who launched the project using contacts from previous projects and the high political interest in assessments aimed at the transport sector.

The assessment was effective in its aims to undertake an integrated assessment of transport-related health effects on children and push the agenda among European decision-makers. The assessment was also successful in using new approaches to assess transport-related health effects (e.g. risk value, willingness to pay, sensitivity analyses, unification of the calculation of health-related external costs).

As noted, not all relevant issues were addressed: for example, the assessment was not able to address equity adequately. This limitation has been recognized by the authors, and hopefully will be considered in more detail soon.

To date, HIA's usefulness as a tool in the decision-making process is virtually unknown to politicians and a wider public in Austria. Traditionally, the political culture in Austria is reluctant to change what is not based on legal reinforcement. Rational decision-making in public health policy is also quite uncommon due to the fact that public health knowledge in general and public health training are in the early stages, behind international standards. However, increased use of HIA in Europe will produce more tools and methodologies as well as its greater acceptance and systematic integration into the decision-making process in Austria.

Our interviewees were all very positive that politicians may soon realize the benefits of HIA as a widely accepted tool by which a policy, programme or project may be judged on its potential health effects and their distribution within a population.

REFERENCES

Arbter K (2004). *SUP – Strategische Umweltprüfung für die Planungspraxis der Zukunft*. Wien, Graz, Neuer Wissenschaftlicher Verlag.

BGBl (2002). Bundesgesetz über die Prüfung der Umweltverträglichkeit (Umweltverträglichkeitsprüfungsgesetz 2000 – UVP-G 2000), BGBl. Nr. 697/1993 idF BGBl. 793/1996, BGBl. I Nr. 89/2000, BGBl. I Nr. 108/2001, BGBl. I Nr. 151/2001 und BGBl. I Nr. 50/2002 (www.umweltbundesamt.at/fileadmin/site/umweltthemen/umweltpolitische/UVP/KonsFassung_UVP-G_2000_idF_50_2002.pdf, accessed 13 August 2006).

Bundesministerium für Land- und Forstwirtschaft Umwelt- und Wasserwirtschaft (BMLFUW) (2004). *Transport-related health effects with a particular focus on children*. Transnational study and workshop series by Austria, France, Malta, the Netherlands, Sweden and Switzerland (www.herry.at/the-pep, accessed 13 August 2006).

Bundesministerium für Land- und Forstwirtschaft Umwelt- und Wasserwirtschaft (BMLFUW) (2005). Gesunde Umwelt für unsere Kinder. WHO Kinder-Umwelt-Gesundheits-Aktionsplan für Europa und Initiativen in Österreich. Wien, Robitschek & Co. 2005. (www.salzburg.gv.at/gesunde_umwelt_fuer_unsere_kinder_-_endversion_05-03-12.pdf, accessed 13 August 2006).

European Centre for Health Policy (1999). *Health impact assessment: main concepts and suggested approach. Gothenburg Consensus Paper*. Brussels, World Health Organization Regional Office for Europe (www.nice.org.uk/media/hiadocs/Gothenburgpaper.pdf, accessed 13 August 2006).

Case study 14

Contributing to a public health culture: health and economic impacts of a health promotion campaign in Denmark

Gabriel Gulis [31]

Introduction

This case study on the health economics and effects of the 6-per-day (Kræftens Bekæmbelse, Syddansk Universitet, Ministeriet for Fødevarer, Landbrug og Fiskeri & Fødevaredirektoratet, 2002) programme has many features (e.g. cost–benefit and policy analyses) of a formal health impact assessment (HIA). It differs from the standard prospective model in that it was initiated by agriculture; taken up by the Cancer Society; conducted with a basic aim of showing the health economic effects of the programme; and was concurrent as well as prospective.

The impact assessment process was led by a steering group that included representatives from the Ministry of Food Production, the Cancer Society and academia. These groups were all involved, and the results were properly disseminated and used to strengthen the campaign and improve intersectoral collaboration. The HIA process proved to be effective for cross-sector exchanges, skills development (knowledge-sharing) and political administration.

This chapter is based on interviews with four of the five members of the assessment's steering committee. Two of the interviewees were responsible for

---

[31] The author declares that neither he nor his unit has conflict of interest regarding the selected case of impact assessment. There was no collaboration between the author and authors of the assessment before this case study.

conducting the assessment. The third was in charge of the assessment on behalf of the initiating organization; and the fourth was involved in the campaign on behalf of the central state administration.

HIA is not well developed in Denmark, especially at national level, so there were not too many cases from which to choose. Other impact assessment methods are used more frequently and are better developed. Risk assessment and life-cycle assessments, for example, focus on risk from chemicals and relate directly to a chemical substance or product (Olsen et al., 2001). Environmental impact assessments (EIAs) have been legal requirements for selected infrastructure projects since 1985, though parliamentary negotiation for major infrastructure projects dates back to the 1880s (Kjellerup, 1999). Economic impact assessments, or rather analyses, have been used since 1980 to assess the cost–benefit aspects of different health-related events (Pedersen, 2005). Health technology assessments followed and were introduced in Denmark around 1984 (Pedersen, 2005).

After detailed literature reviews, two studies were selected for inclusion in the effectiveness of HIA project: the 6-per-day (*6 om dagen*) case and a case study of a diesel particle filter effectiveness assessment. The latter represents an analytical life-cycle assessment based on a single product. The choice of the 6-per-day assessment was rather simple as it contains the main elements to qualify as an HIA. There was a formal steering group; public sector (Cancer Society, Heart Association) and decision-makers' (ministries, national boards) involvement; a huge element of intersectoral collaboration; and a focus on economic and health effects (impacts of the programme).

The first part of this chapter describes briefly the national HIA context in Denmark. The second analyses the execution of the selected study and the third discusses the effectiveness of the assessment. The chapter concludes with the main findings. Information is based on the experiences gathered through individual interviews with participants in the assessment.

Profiling the HIA within Denmark

At the time of the selected assessment (1999–2001) HIA had not formally been introduced on a national level in Denmark. An 18-month review by the National Institute of Public Health produced the first and, until now, only report analysing HIA in Denmark (Bistrup & Kamper-Jørgensen, 2005). This was published in 2004 and introduced the term into the national level of policy- and decision-making.

Based on the growing evidence from international epidemiology literature and the interests of different production associations and institutions, in 1998 and 1999 the Ministry of Food Production and the Danish Cancer Society decided to organize a nationwide campaign to increase fruit and vegetable consumption. The Danish Cancer Society led this process and, although the campaign had an obvious positive impact on health, chose to use this opportunity to undertake an assessment process. One of the interviewees explained the twin aims:

> We wanted to get clear data, clear evidence that there is an important health effect of increased fruit and vegetable consumption which can lead to health care savings and we also wanted to move the issue higher on political agenda. Therefore we initiated this intersectoral assessment process …

The decision to conduct the 6-per-day campaign was made in 1999 and the campaign was launched in 2001. Initially the impact assessment was not a part of the decision-making process – there was no pending decision related to this assessment. It was conducted in parallel with the development and preparation of the campaign; as the interviewee stated above, it aimed to increase the agenda on a political level. However, another challenge linked to the assessment process was described by a second interviewee: " … our aim was to test in practice our ability to conduct an assessment project with truly intersectoral participation … "

These are important facts to recognize when trying to profile the selected assessment case study within the country. The campaign was national and expected to have a positive influence on the consumption of fruit and vegetables, producing health gains and economic savings related to health-care use. Business, agriculture, nongovernmental organization (NGO) and academic sectors were equally interested in the achievements of the campaign and results of the assessment process.

At the time of the assessment no formal model could be followed as HIA was neither formally implemented nor introduced by Danish scientific literature. Denmark uses the translation of the HIA definition in the Gothenburg consensus paper (European Centre for Health Policy, 1999) and the 6-per-day assessment matches this. The clearly defined aim of the assessment was to assess future health impacts of a recent policy (campaign). Intersectoral participation was not only a method, but also a specific objective of the assessment. It was guided by a multisectoral steering group and scoping, risk assessment and reporting were completed.

The initial assessment process was stimulated by interest from representatives of agriculture, business and the Cancer Society. This interest replaces the formal screening in assessment. The assessment case (the health impact of the

6-per-day campaign) is considered a research project. The programme was launched concurrently with the assessment and in this case no formal decision-making was expected. As with the programme, the assessment was conducted on the national level.

The Ministry of Food Production (*Ministeriet for Fødevare, Landbrug og Fiskeri*), Danish Cancer Society (*Kræftens Bekæmbelse*), and The University of Southern Denmark (*Syddansk Universitet*) were key actors and stakeholders in the assessment process. Other important players were the Danish Fitness and Nutrition Council (*Motions- og Ernæringsradet*), National Consumer Agency (*Forbrugerstyrelsen*), Garden Centres Sales and Marketing Committee (*Gartneribrugets afsætningsudvalg*), Danish Fruit, Vegetable and Potato Board (*Forskningsforeningen for Frugt, Gront og Kartofler*), Danish Veterinary and Food Administration (*Fødevarestyrelsen*), Danish Heart Association (*Hjerteforeningen*), and the National Board of Health (*Sundhedsstyrelsen*).

The Ministry of Food Production was one of the key initiators of the campaign and assessment and co-funded the assessment process. The Danish Cancer Society was the main moving force, initiator and sponsor of the process. The Centre of Advanced Economic Studies, University of Southern Denmark, carried out the assessment. Results were disseminated in a one-day seminar at the Danish Parliament, so the stakeholder role of other Danish government ministries and the Parliament itself has been recognized and acknowledged.

The assessment's steering group met five times during the two-year assessment process. It comprised representatives of the Danish Cancer Society (chairperson, epidemiologist and a nutrition epidemiologist), two representatives of the Ministry of Food Production (specialists on cardiovascular disease prevention), a statistician and the two researchers from University of Southern Denmark who carried out the analysis. The assessment was purely a research project so there was no public representative in the steering group.

Aims of the HIA and dimensions of effectiveness

The aims of the assessment were as stated by the interviewees:

- to show the 6-per-day campaign's effectiveness as a health promotion campaign
- to bring this issue to the political agenda
- to test a truly intersectoral (multi-stakeholder) collaboration.

Using a cohort model, the intention of the HIA was to analyse changes in life expectancy and how these would alter the influence of health-care spending (Sørensen, 1999). The results were expected to inform politicians with the aim of increasing the use of similar tools for cost–benefit analyses of health promotions, general health intervention policies, campaigns and so on.

The assessment has shown clear benefits of the campaign in terms of an increase in life expectancy. However, it failed to show health–economic benefits. The assessment fulfilled its second aim to inform politicians. A one-day workshop, with good mediation and participation, was conducted at the end of the assessment process at the national parliament (*Folketinget*) and at government level.

The assessment addressed predominantly the environmental and social determinants of health; health care issues such as determinants of health were addressed to some extent.

Regarding the aims of the assessment, interviewees focused on the health and community dimensions of effectiveness. Equity-related issues were not addressed; a cohort based on a 20% random sample of the Danish population served as the basis for the analysis, sampled from general Danish population and health databases (Sørensen, 1999). This cohort was not divided further by social or any other factors and the equity issue was not addressed specifically. Consequently, the equity dimension of the assessment's effectiveness has not been discussed.

Interviewees reported that although the assessment process did not affect decisions concerning effects on health it substantially increased politicians' (health and non-health) awareness of health promotion, nutrition and public health in general. As one interviewee stated: "After the assessment process and presentation of results the Minister (of Food Production) herself always referred to the report as a successful one … ". Moreover, participation in the assessment work greatly increased health professionals' ability to argue, both within and outside the health sector, on matters related to health promotion and disease prevention. One of the interviewees reported: "I felt (after assessment process) much more empowered, much more confident in discussions with colleagues, medical doctors, in matters of importance of health promotion, disease prevention … " In summary, the interviewees agreed upon general health effectiveness for the assessment process.

No direct measure of community effectiveness is implied in the assessment process and its results. However, steering group members claimed important administrative and political effectiveness. Political interest and willingness to support similar assessment procedures were clearly articulated by politicians and government ministers during and after the final presentation of the assessment.

Trust in the possibility of conducting a successful and truly intersectoral, multi-stakeholder collaboration has increased greatly. One interviewee commented: "I would never before believe that we can so nicely and fruitfully collaborate with economists on health issues."

In the long-term, these factors are likely to have positive impacts on introducing impact assessment procedures and the culture of multi-stakeholder collaboration into the community. As we considered community effectiveness based on the concept of empowerment, there seems to be an important community effectiveness element in this assessment process. This is best defined not as direct community effectiveness, but rather as a secondary work culture that builds effectiveness within the community (e.g. participatory collaborative work and public health culture) – a culture of empowerment. This type of community effectiveness has also been highlighted in a Danish report dealing with the possibilities of cross-sector collaboration (DEA & Djøf, 2005).

Process, input and context of HIA

This section presents an analysis of how the process of conducting the HIA corresponds or interrelates with the decision-making process and community dynamics. For analytical purposes, three elements are distinguished: process, input and context.

Process

The assessment process was not linked to a pending decision therefore it is not possible to analyse it from a policy-cycle perspective. However, two points are important in terms of Denmark's policy cycle. Firstly, Denmark is a largely decentralized country where important decisions are made at local and regional levels. Successful implementation of an HIA and its links to policy cycles are highly dependent on raising public-health awareness among politicians, decision-makers and the public at each level of decision-making. Interviewees emphasized the assessment's great success in achieving this. Secondly, although interviewees did not anticipate major controversies about the introduction of the HIA, they agreed that legal requirement of impact assessment procedures would ensure that they are used more frequently.

As described and argued earlier, no formal HIA model was followed. However, the main stages of methodology such as scoping, assessment and reporting were clearly completed.

As agreed in scoping, a cohort based on a 20% random sample of the Danish population was used for the risk assessment calculation. In this case the risk assessment focused on the health and health–economic gains related to the subject of assessment, rather than analysis and assessment of risks. The broader socioeconomic model of health was employed. The interviewees recognized that good health and economic statistics for Denmark were important and strong enablers for conducting and completing the assessment process.

Input

Inputs are defined as who takes the lead and who directs the HIA. In the 6-per-day assessment all possible inputs played a significant role. Although it had no political representative on the steering group, the Ministry of Food Production played a key role in launching and conducting the assessment. It supported the process and, most importantly, participated actively in the presentation and further mediation of results and the assessment process.

There is no legal input regarding HIA in Denmark, i.e. no "owner" as such, but administrative input was initiated and supported strongly by the Danish Cancer Society, who took over this role. Although less visible, there was clear and substantial community input from the different agricultural and business associations that participated in the initiation of the assessment. They created a specific community by sharing common interests and were strongly supportive in this assessment process. None of the participants were legally obliged to participate in the assessment.

It is possible to conclude that legal input is unnecessary if all other inputs are present and collaborating well. Although not required by statute, an HIA process that is interdisciplinary and based on values such as participation, public involvement, democracy (in the 6-per-day case: from the agricultural to the health sector, from farmers to the Minister) and the ethical use of evidence (data from existing databases and literature) could be effective in influencing the future impacts of decisions.

Context

As the interviewees concluded, the main effectiveness of the assessment is an increased belief in the strength of interdisciplinary, multi-stakeholder work and the ability for health promotion and disease prevention to make a difference and increase public health culture in Denmark. They explicitly asked for more, and similar, impact assessments and expressed their willingness to support them. They also mentioned the concept of public health and health promotion as a relatively new development in Denmark and a possible strong enabler for future implementation of HIAs.

After a long preparation period, a new state- and local-level administration model was implemented recently in Denmark. The so-called "structure reform" (Indenrigs- og Sundhedsministreriet, 2004) presents new municipalities with the challenge of responsibility for health promotion and public health and opens a new window of opportunity for HIA.

Each of the interviewees mentioned statutory implementation of HIA as a likely strong enabler but there is no clear picture of how this should be done.

The interviewees also mentioned another important contextual issue: the availability of data. Denmark has many well-managed database resources for both determinants of health and health outcomes. Availability of these data resources is seen as a clear enabler for impact assessment techniques.

Conclusion

The presented assessment was completed under rather atypical circumstances. It is a research case, not linked to a pending decision, concurrent in timing and does not follow a formal methodology. Nevertheless it shows great health and community effectiveness (production of new knowledge, intersectoral collaboration and the ability to argue health-promotion and disease-prevention issues). The assessment has shown the need for, and the value of, good and available data; without these the assessment would not have been possible.

Frequently, HIAs focus on changes in the determinants of health. This case study shows that HIA might not only impact on direct health, community or equity but also contribute to a long-term public health culture.

The large structural change in the country's administration offers more opportunities for HIA. The reforms have granted the new municipalities important responsibilities for health promotion and public health, and they are searching for new working methods and skilled personnel. Conversely, until recently there was little change at the national level.

REFERENCES

Bistrup ML & Kamper-Jørgensen F (2005). *Sundhedskonsekvensvurderinger: koncept, perspektiver, anvendelse i stat, amter og kommuner [Health impact assessments: concepts, perspectives, application by government, regions, and municipalities]*. Copenhagen, The Government Institute of Public Health.

DEA & Djøf (2005). *Danmarks erhvervsforskningsbarometer: Sådan samarbejder virksomheder og universiteter [The Danish occupational research barometer: this is how companies and universities coorporate].* Copenhagen, DEA (http://www.dea.nu/log/dea/library/ Danmarks%20Erhvervsforskningsbarometer%202005.pdf, accessed 22 December 2005).

European Centre for Health Policy (1999). *Health impact assessment: main concepts and suggested approach. Gothenburg consensus paper.* Brussels, WHO Regional Office for Europe (http://www.euro.who.int/document/PAE/Gothenburgpaper.pdf, accessed 15 June 2006).

Indenrigs- og Sundhedsministreriet (2004) [Danish Ministry of the Interior and Health]. *Kommunalreformen – De politiske aftaler [The municipal reform – the political agreements].* Copenhagen, Ministry of the Interior and Health (http://www.im.dk/publikationer/komreform_politiske_aft/html/87-7601-201-8.pdf, accessed 27 March 2006).

Kjellerup U (1999). Legal problems in Danish EIA – the Oeresund case. *Journal of Environmental Assessment, Policy and Management,* 1(1):131–149.

Olsen SI, et al. (2001). Life cycle impact assessment and risk assessment of chemicals – a methodological comparison. *Environmental Impact Assessment Review,* 21:385–404.

Pedersen KM (2005). *Sundhedspolitik: Beslutningsgrundlag, beslutningstagen og beslutninger i sundhedsvæsnet [Health policy: basis for decisions, decision-making, and decisions in health care].* Odense, Syddansk Universitetsforlag [University of Southern Denmark publishers].

Sørensen J (1999). *Vurdering af de sundhedsøkonomiske konsekvenser ved et øget indtag af frugt og grønsager [Valuation of the health economic consequenses of an increase intake of fruit and vegetables].* Odense, Cast – SDU.

Kræftens Bekæmbelse, Syddansk Universitet, Ministeriet for fødevarer, landbrug og fiskeri & Fødevaredirektoratet (2002) [Kræftens Bekæmbelse, University of Southern Denmark, The Danish Ministry of Food, Agriculture and Fishing & The Directory of Foods]. *6 om dagen: Sundhedsmæssige og sundhedsøkonomiske konsekvenser [6-a-day: Health and Health Economic consequenses].*

Case study 15

Removing hurdles towards HIA: pilot project of an obstacle-free environment in Hungary

Edit Eke [32]

Introduction

This pilot study was the first intended health impact assessment (HIA) in Hungary. While it did not influence any pending decision, its pioneer role was an important factor for selection in this case study. The study benefited crucially from the commitment of those willing to support and contribute to it.

HIA of an obstacle-free environment was a national-level pilot project with two central aims. The first was to examine how success or failure to ensure an obstacle-free environment in public buildings and workplaces affects the health and quality of life of people with disabilities, their carers and families. The second aim was to carry out the first Hungarian HIA study in order to test its methodology and to develop additional proposals regarding its further introduction and legitimacy.

The pilot project faced several challenges as it introduced a previously unknown approach and type of assessment into the country. Significantly, political changes interrupted the project's continuity (including its high-level health policy support) through changes in personnel, health policy agenda and priorities.

[32] Neither the author nor the institute was involved in the presented HIA pilot project. The institute and the author dealt with this study for research purposes as partners in the effectiveness of HIA project. Acknowledgements: the author would like to thank the generous support of the following people. Margit Ohr (project leader, National Institute for Health Development (NIHD)), Lilla Vető (project team member, NIHD), Lajos Hegedűs (assigned project expert, President of the National Federation of Disabled Persons' Associations) and Ágnes Ratalics (senior consultant, Ministry of Health) – all of whom kindly offered their knowledge, expertise and experiences in the field of HIA. This greatly supported the work.

This chapter profiles the study and its effectiveness based on the available literature, documents and information, including one partial interview (with the project leader) and two full interviews (with a key member of the project team and with the President of the National Federation of Disabled Persons' Associations).

HIA became an important issue with Hungary's accession to the EU (1 May 2004). The Hungarian equivalent of HIA is *egészséghatás vizsgálat* (EHV) and the domestic definition of HIA is:

> Assessment of impacts on health is the combined use of such proceedings, methods and means that are appropriate to assess the effects of professional policies, programmes and projects on the health of the population and to assess the distribution of these effects in the society (Ohr & Vető, 2005).

This chapter is presented in four sections. The first profiles the HIA, stressing some specific context issues. The second concentrates on the aims of the study and the dimension of effectiveness. The third is about the process, input and context of the HIA, and the last section presents a conclusion.

Profiling the HIA pilot project

Legal situation

Legal, operative policy documents cover HIA, its role and importance. The ten-year national public health programme accepted in 2004 outlined the main directions of development for the health of the population, health care and related issues in Hungary. But the strategic and practical implementations of HIA, particularly enforcement of the laws that ensure that these requirements are fulfilled and monitored, are either missing or not followed. However, appropriate use and interpretation of HIA term have been increasing in the past few years.

Specific background information and context

In July 2003, the Department of Health Impact Assessment (DHIA) was established at the National Institute for Health Development (NIHD), part of the National Public Health and Medical Officer Service. The project leader came from NIHD and has a strong personal interest in HIA. She completed relevant training at IMPACT in Liverpool, and has held international and policy fellowship positions where research activity focused on HIA – namely, working with the Open Society Institute on *Moving from research to practice in the policy process: design and delivery of health impact assessment pilot project.*

In 2004 the NIHD published an issue in a series (Kishegyi & Makara, 2004), dedicated to HIA.

The project leader's Hungarian policy mentor was the Political Secretary of the Ministry of Health, Social and Family Affairs. In autumn 2003, he was appointed Minister of Health, Social and Family Affairs. The project leader acknowledged the Minister's strong interest in, and commitment to, HIA and its introduction in Hungary.

In 2003, an informal HIA workshop was organized to introduce the results of ongoing research and discuss the supporting and obstructing factors. It was also intended to choose the theme of a potential national pilot study. According to the interviewees, it was a political intention and decision to conduct a national-level HIA pilot study. There was no pending decision; the relating law was accepted already. As one interviewee stressed, the HIA pilot study was "unexpected", but they were happy to have that option.

In spring 2004, the Minister of Health, Social and Family Affairs decided on the theme of the national pilot study – disability affairs. In June 2004, NIHD and the Ministry of Health, Social and Family Affairs entered into a contract for a national HIA pilot study; NIHD was in charge of coordination. The planned time frame was September 2004 to December 2005. The theme was the health assessment of the obstacle-free environment. All interviewees stressed that this was interpreted with broad meaning and understanding and used in a comprehensive way: no obstacle to access information, buildings, services, and so on. Physical accessibility was considered as one component of the obstacle-free environment. Health determinants were examined in their complexity. The pilot study was concerned with six sectors of the HIA theme: education, employment, health care, social issues, legal environment and economic impacts.

In 2003, it was estimated that an obstacle-free environment was ensured in 20–30% of all public buildings at national level. A questionnaire survey of health-care institutions showed that only 21% were obstacle-free.

The rights of disabled people and the principle of equality guaranteed for them are defined by Law 1998/XXVI. In February 2004, the Ministry of Health, Social and Family Affairs submitted several proposals to modify different laws concerning social and health issues, including Law 1998/XXVI. The submission of changes to the 1998 law and the start of HIA activities were concurrent. Law 1998/XXVI and the attached enforcement resolution, Resolution 100/1999 (XII.10) OGY of the National Assembly, fixed a deadline for 1 January 2005 for creating an obstacle-free environment in all public buildings. This deadline was not met and this remains a sensitive issue, especially politically.

The HIA pilot project did not influence the law as this was passed even before the formation of any ideas for the HIA. Yet it is obvious that an obstacle-free environment has great effects on health aspects for affected population groups. The HIA was to provide decision-makers with adequate information "about the situation of disabled people and the development of obstacle-free environment thus facilitating the validation of interests defined by law" (Ohr, 2005).

One interviewee, President of the National Federation of Disabled Persons' Associations, said he did not know what factors determined the realization and theme of the HIA but felt the knowledge, expertise, commitment and enthusiasm of the project leader was essential. She wanted to use her international experience to introduce HIA in Hungary where it was "totally new" and found strong supporters, in decision-making positions, to be able to do this. Hungary joined the EU in May 2004, the 'Year of People with Disabilities', optimal for both the timing and the theme of the HIA pilot study. HIA literacy was generally low among the invited and then assigned professionals (experts in their own fields).

Aims of the HIA

The principal aim of the obstacle-free environment HIA pilot project was to examine:

> … how the fulfilment or failure of ensuring obstacle-free environment in public buildings and workplaces affects the health and quality of life of people with disabilities, their carers and families. The assessment does not include private service providers (hotels, banks …) (Ohr, 2005).

Another was "to carry out the first Hungarian HIA in order to test its methodology and to develop additional proposals regarding its further introduction and legitimacy" (Ohr, 2005).

One of the interviewees noted the aim to introduce accountability, existing alongside a law, and providing evidence of its reality and importance. Also, the option of a nationwide HIA was intended to call attention to the crucial role of impact assessments and influence general thinking about them.

Dimensions of effectiveness

General effectiveness

Based on the available information and the interviewees' opinions, the pilot study did not achieve its original specific aims but had some mainly opportunistic effects. Its main direct effect was to raise some awareness of the situation of people with disabilities and the environmental challenges they face. Also it supported the endeavour to understand the complexity and components of an obstacle-free environment and what an HIA study means. These effects were partly due to the media attention attracted by the theme.

One of the interviewees noted that the pilot project had no direct influence on the situation of people with disabilities: "As it was not published and available for the public, nobody except the persons who were included has knowledge about this HIA pilot study". However, he identified some indirect, opportunistic effect as other involved, assigned experts' views of disability affairs had changed completely in the course of the work:

> I had significant influence on the thinking of those people as they simply did not have any knowledge of disability affairs. They were interested and asked me in order to clarify their own approach to these affairs. Thus, they know much more about it now. Some of them read our materials, too. I consider the increase of interest and change of approach of some people to be the use of the work. The study was effective via the people who were involved in the project.

This interviewee was sorry that there was no link to the "New National Programme of Disability Affairs 2007–2013", and felt that at least the existing, incomplete parts of the report and the experiences of the pilot study should have been used more effectively in new health policy materials: "It could have been included as a part of these documents. Now, even the completed parts of the report may be lost forever, as the step to call attention to it and put it forward for further use – in its state as not fully completed – did not happen." He felt that an effect could have been expected only if the decision-makers had received information about the pilot study and its result. Consequently they could have realized what positive effects the obstacle-free environment can ensure not only for the life of people with disabilities, but also for the whole society. As it was missed, he thinks that the crucial importance of such an approach for the health of each person, including people with disabilities, did not get across at all.

Health effectiveness

The interviewees did not identify direct health effectiveness. They felt the pilot study highlighted an issue: the situation for people with disabilities and the importance of ensuring an obstacle-free environment. Thus some indirect general health effectiveness was achieved.

Also, the project raised some awareness of HIA among health-policy advisers and decision-makers, politicians, health and other professionals and the general population. This can be taken as an opportunistic health effectiveness.

Equity effectiveness

Two interviewees considered that the HIA pilot study not only drew attention to equity issues among people with disabilities and the rest of the society, but also brought equity (equal judgement and treatment) for population groups with different disabilities into consideration among policy-makers, affected groups and society. Thus it had moderate general equity effectiveness.

Community effectiveness

This pilot study was conceived as a national project but one interviewee said that it was highly centralized to the capital – most people involved, including professionals and other stakeholders, lived and worked in Budapest. No other regional centre and/or organization had a direct active role in the project. The disproportionate number of people from the capital who participated in the study draws further attention to the aspect of equity and community effectiveness as more access and participation were required across sectors in society.

Representatives of the affected communities in leading positions were involved. As far as can be judged, members of these organizations did not receive much information about the HIA pilot study, but one interviewee reported that they were "happy". This was mainly because the theme of the HIA reflected and highlighted issues of importance to people with disabilities. Generally the HIA itself made no material difference for them but it was considered to have gathered general community support by drawing society's attention to the needs of those with disabilities.

Other dimensions of effectiveness

The pilot study introduced HIA methodology, and helped to raise awareness of HIA's role. It led to the creation of HIA methodology and policy guidelines in the Hungarian language as one chapter of the final report (even if it has not been published yet). The pilot study contributed to further, in-depth and strategic consideration and inclusion of HIA in policy documents. It highlighted the fact that existing methods, methodologies, and strategies intended to include HIA in decision-making processes must be critically revised and/or completed with adequate means to make HIA work in practice. This includes appropriate and sustainable capacity and resource development, effective coordination, human-resource training, control, and so on. It highlighted the shortage and/or inadequate level of HIA understanding and expertise at professional level and in general. It drew attention to the necessity for high-level specific training required to complete any HIA successfully.

The pilot study also drew attention to affected population groups at professional levels, among the affected population groups themselves and throughout society, and highlighted the existing inequities and failure of attempts to achieve significant improvement.

The pilot study attracted media attention towards disability affairs and the HIA itself. However, one interviewee noted that in their opinion the HIA, its importance and the pilot study itself received much less attention and lacked a good introduction of its theme. The media itself did not really understand the issue and did not really care; the HIA was not in focus. The interviewee involved in disability affairs said he could not judge the media attention as "from inside" it made no difference.

One interviewee noted good effectiveness for project management and its commission in the preparation phase. The experts had good and inspiring connections with each other and the project team. Their work was effective.

Input, process and context of the HIA pilot project

Input

The Johan Béla National Programme for the Decade of Health was accepted in April 2003. A small sum in its budget was earmarked to organize a conference and prepare and run a national HIA pilot project. An HIA conference was organized in autumn 2004. All ministers and members of the Health Committee of the National Assembly were invited and many stakeholders and key players participated. The conference programme included a workshop on behalf of the European Commission in which several Hungarian and some European health politicians participated. Their important decision-making positions and commitment to HIA and its introduction in Hungary were evaluated by the interviewees to be crucial to the realization and development of HIA activities and the pilot project.

Hungary's leading role in coordinating central eastern-European HIA was enhanced. The project leader emphasized that she preferred regular HIA training to organizing and hosting a conference. Among several reasons for the failure of her suggestion, it was important that she was not in a position with adequate political and professional power to be able to validate it. Beyond that, the financial background did not make it possible to realize both the training and the conference, which would have been optimal. But the conference provided a well-arranged start: an introductory event for the main stakeholders and experts. It was very successful, but later experiences in the project stressed the vital importance of high-level professional HIA training.

The first project meeting was organized after the conference and served as the opening workshop. Altogether 44 stakeholders and experts were invited and involved in the preparation process "from all relevant parts of disability affairs" (Ohr, 2005).

The NIHD contracted six experts to participate in the National HIA Pilot Study, develop professional guidelines and prepare the relevant evaluations and reports. This team grew to eight members by including two of the project team from NIHD as experts. A core project team at NIHD coordinated and managed the process and carried out the study. The team members did not belong to the same department (DHIA) and comprised: the project leader (at NIHD from 1994; became head of the DHIA in 2003); a social politician who was an expert on disability affairs and relating obstacle-free environmental issues (also participated in the preparation of the National Programme of Disability Affairs); an economist and a political scientist.

The HIA's financial background has been mentioned. The ensured sum was shared between the conference and the pilot project. Members of the core team were NIHD employees. The NIHD is a public institution, funded out of the state budget.

The pilot project time frame was September 2004 to July 2005. Interviewees indicated that the driving force behind the tight time frame and deadline was provided by the tight time constraint on the ensured money. The final deadline of the project was modified to December 2005 in the course of the HIA. The report of the study was delivered to the Ministry of Health although some parts of the final report are still pending. The report has not yet been published and/or discussed in public. We do not have information regarding its professional and/or inner distribution and use in the Ministry of Health.

One interviewee (the project leader) said that the project's overall quality could and should be much better. More work is needed to finalize it, but no future resources are ensured. This interviewee gave the evaluation that this deficiency mostly is due to the lack of adequate and real understanding and knowledge of HIA, even among professional experts, and this is beyond what could have been influenced throughout the project and its aftermath.

This view is supported by interviewees' remarks that most of the assigned professionals lacked real HIA knowledge and understanding. Two interviewees (project team members) considered that they had found it difficult to conform to the theme of the HIA as many of them were "stuck" in their own positions and interests. A varying level of commitment and openness to HIA produced difficult consequences and one weak point of the pilot study.

The third interviewee said he did not have previous knowledge of HIA: "It was new for all of us. It was not a known thing." Following his appointment he studied the issue in the literature and developed his knowledge. His orientation was helped further by talking about HIA with partner associations at an international level (European Disability Forum). Also he stressed that the project leader and her team had a highly professional approach to HIA and provided training and help whenever it was required throughout the project. It was the individual responsibility of the assigned experts if, and to what extent, they looked further into the issue.

Although most project participants had little or no previous knowledge of HIA, most were committed and enthusiastic, ready to develop their knowledge and skills and perform project work to their best ability. They discussed the potential themes in the given framework, decided the final theme and identified and chose experts. Also, they considered topics such as education and training, integrated care and employment.

The final choice of the theme – HIA of an obstacle-free environment – was supported strongly by its links to other considered issues, and its expected positive effects on all fields. It was a common denominator. One interviewee perceived a gradual formation of the approach to, and interpretation of, "obstacle-free environment". It started with the literal physical approach and developed into equal accessibility for all, binding it further to the "design for all" principle. As with other participants he joined the project when there was "broad definition" of the decisions of the national HIA pilot study and its theme, but the definitive theme had not been identified. This interviewee explains the course of the work as represented by the points listed here.

1 Theme definition.
2 Orientations: what will be the content?
3 Discussion of experts' suggestions; decision regarding the task assignments and responsibility, discussion and forming of the structure of the HIA pilot study.
4 Discussion and evaluation of the pending drafts, following individual work of the experts, accompanied by e-mail correspondence with other experts and the inner project team at NIHD. Deadline for the final drafts for discussion was originally June 2005 but postponed to August 2005. This project meeting took place in August 2005.
5 Finalization of the materials.

According to this interviewee, his work ended here. His last contact was an e-mail feedback from the project leader notifying him about the acceptance of the professional work (step six as acceptance of final materials). He saw neither the final report (step seven, the final stage of the process) nor any final parts from other experts; only drafts from other experts during the working period – partly for review, partly to avoid duplication. He had no information about the acceptance of the final report and/or if any relating publications have been issued. "The whole thing was not closed, summarized, pulled together. There was not a complete material at the end of it."

The large, closing workshop did not take place. It was planned for the first quarter of 2005 in order to evaluate the results of professional work, form conclusions and recommendations, and produce a comprehensive study that summarized all results. It is not fully understood why this meeting was not held but it seems to have been influenced by changes to wider political relations related to health care, including personnel issues; and problems with inadequate levels of understanding and professional knowledge of HIA among the experts.

Process

As mentioned earlier, the decision to conduct a national-level HIA pilot study and the choice of field on which it was based were politically driven in 2004. No decision was pending.

Although screening and scoping were simultaneous, screening was problematic because of the special contexts described above. One of the interviewees reported that scoping was correct. Further HIA stages, including appraisal, recommendation, decision-making, ongoing evaluation and monitoring, were either not carried out or only partially carried out, owing largely to the special characteristics of this HIA project, including the lack of any pending decision and the interruption of the project.

The HIA was interpreted in accordance with the Gothenburg consensus (European Centre for Health Policy, 1999). No specific model was used, and the project followed information on the methodology and model of several national HIA projects in other countries. No formal HIA model in practice had been introduced and used in the country.

The HIA's steering group included the participating experts and colleagues of the core project team, completed by the director of the NIHD. It was neither formal nor fixed on paper and did not hold regular formal meetings as a steering group. However, as interviewees mentioned, most of these people worked closely together every day and the project had a very tight time frame.

According to all interviewees it was intended to include and use the report and its results in several health and/or social policy documents: for example, in the New National Programme of Disability Affairs 2007–2013; the Health Policy Development Concept Note, to the decrees and resolution acts of the Johan Béla National Programme for the Decade of Health; and even in the relevant parts of the National Development Plan (known as The New Hungary Development Plan). Originally it was planned that the pilot study and its final report would have played an important role in health policy, and to implement HIA in all policies.

It was intended to consider the economic impacts of the cost of creating an obstacle-free environment and the direct and indirect economic consequences and benefits of its realization. The latter proved too difficult to cover fully because of a shortage of data and valid estimations. One interviewee mentioned that "sport, culture and leisure activities" were going to be included, but finally they were not. Six experts outside the project team (in which two experts covered the methodological section) were assigned and contracted. Each was responsible for one of the sections.

The HIA project team met regularly with the experts' group, three to four times during the project, and provided support and feedback. Also, they were the first reviewers of the experts' documents. As the contracting party, the Ministry of Health received electronic and paper drafts of the HIA report. Interviewees said that they had no further influence on events and have no knowledge if and how the document was evaluated and used.

Context

It is important to summarize how the interviewees evaluated the main driving force behind the national HIA pilot study. The personal enthusiasm and professional expertise of a few people met with indirect political support. Although this received real action and direct support from the political level at an "optimal" moment in a favourable political situation, later the continuity and follow-up of the HIA were missing at administrative and political levels. The interviewees did not experience any real interest, and did not have any feed-back about the project.

Two interviewees said that there is no legal background or force to HIA in Hungary. Generally, health is not an issue that is taken into account and there is no public health culture. One interviewee said that HIA cannot be an issue of political controversy as politicians do not have adequate knowledge about it; there is a lack of HIA knowledge even at decision-makers' level. Another interviewee had the opinion that some moderate favourable changes occurred at least among some politicians. All interviewees stressed that suitable training and HIA capacity development, including human resources, are essential in order to proceed. One interviewee added that motivation, international pressure and favourable change in the general approach towards HIA, especially at health-policy level, could help greatly in the future.

Conclusion

Specific conclusions of this HIA pilot study

The interviewees concluded the points listed here:

- HIA expertise and capacity are scarce in Hungary. There is a need to develop capacities and high-level training.

- The pilot study was too expansive – intending to cover all types of disability and all factors of an obstacle-free environment. The focus should have been much narrower, more well defined and realistic, for both the issues covered and the specific aspects to study.

- Experiments in other countries can be very helpful, but critical adaptation is vital to take account of special characteristics.

- The importance and essence of HIA did not "get through", despite media attention.

- Political factors are especially important and have deep influences on such activity and its success in Hungary.

General conclusions regarding HIA in Hungary

There has been much emphasis on this issue. More and more health policies, policy-makers and other politicians consider HIA and refer to the necessity for well-planned and well-managed HIAs and their optimal role in decision-making processes. Even so, the current situation is not adequate.

While there is commitment, existing strategic decisions and a legal background, at present it can be stated that Hungary has:

- no adequate or effective HIA organization or suitable personnel (although NIHD has a department dedicated to HIA);

- no suitable financing, regular or allocated money for HIA and related activities;

- no clear and transparent national, declared and accepted policy and/or strategy to introduce and manage HIA, or spread existing information and achievements;

- not enough training capacities and expertise. Similar to at professional and political levels, and in society, awareness and real knowledge of HIA are insufficient.

There is a strong and declared commitment to HIA on the part of health policy and political decision-making. Yet so far the overall impression is that HIA and its practice have depended largely on the strong personal commitment of some individuals, and their options to influence any HIA-related decision and money allocation. However, the last comprehensive professional health policy document – the Health Policy Development Concept Note – dedicated several passages to HIA. It clearly identified HIA as a very important issue that deserves and needs priority (Egészségügyi Fejlesztéspolitikai Koncepció, 2005). This approach and interpretation partly may be due to the first national-level HIA Pilot Study, although there is no direct evidence for this.

REFERENCES

Egészségügyi Fejlesztéspolitikai Koncepció (2005). *Health policy development concept note 31/08/2005.* Budapest, Ministry of Health (http://www.eum.hu/index.php?akt_menu=3300, accessed 6 September 2005).

European Centre for Health Policy (1999). *Health impact assessment: main concepts and suggested approaches. Gothenburg consensus paper.* Brussels, WHO Regional Office for Europe (http://www.euro.who.int/document/PAE/Gothenburgpaper.pdf, accessed 15 June 2006).

Kishegyi J, Makara, P eds (2004). Az egészséghatás vizsgálat. [The Health Impact Assessment]. *Egészségfejlesztési Módszertani Füzetek [Methodological Booklets of Health Development]*, 7:74 (http://www.oefi.hu/modszert.htm, accessed 24 May 2005).

Law 1998 XXVI (1998). évi XXVI *törvény a fogyatékos személyek jogairól és esélyegyenlőségük biztosításáról [Act No. XXVI on provision of the rights of persons living with disability and guarantee the principle of equality for them].* Magyar Közlöny (Hungarian Gazette) (http://www.meoszinfo.hu/index_23_02.php, accessed 5 October 2006).

Ohr M (2005). *Egészséghatás vizsgálat az akadálymentesítésről [Health impact assessment study of obstacle-free environment].* Budapest, National Institute for Health Development (http://www.oefi.hu/, accessed 9 May 2005).

Ohr M, Vető L (2005). *Egészséghatás vizsgálat modellkísérlet: módszertani fejezet, Országos Egészségfejlesztési Intézet [HIA pilot project: chapter on methodology].* Budapest, National Institute for Health Development.
[Please note, this is one chapter of the study report that has not been published yet, and there is no official English translation.]

Resolution 100/1999 (XII.10) (1999). *Országgyűlési Határozat az Országos Fogyatékosügyi Programró [Resolution of the National Assembly No. 100/1999 on the National Programme of Disability Affairs].* Magyar Közlöny (Hungarian Gazette) (http://www.fogyatekosugy.hu/, accessed 1 August 2006).

Resolution 46/2003 (2003). *Az egészség évtizedének Johan Béla Nemzeti Programjáról szóló 46/2003 (IV.16) OGY határozat [Resolution of the National Assembly No. 46/2003 (IV.16) OGY on the Johan Béla National Programme for the Decade of Health].* Magyar Közlöny (Hungarian Gazette) (http://www.eum.hu/index.php?akt_menu=3538, accessed 12 November 2004).

Case study 16

Traffic and transport at the local level: capacity building for HIA in Ireland

Teresa Lavin and Owen Metcalfe

Introduction

The National Health Strategy (Department of Health and Children, 2001) identified health impact assessment (HIA) as an important process by which to achieve the goal of improved population health. Since then the Institute of Public Health has worked on a programme to develop HIA as part of public policy.

This case study reviews a comprehensive HIA of traffic and transport at local level. This was retrospective therefore there was no pending decision to be influenced. However, it was one of the first HIAs to be conducted in Ireland and is a good example of using available resources to test HIA methodology in practice. Furthermore it demonstrates how the findings of this process can be used to influence future development. In addition, it highlights the opportunities and barriers for different sectors working together at the local level on an issue which was strongly influenced by plans and policies at a much wider level.

The information for this case study is based on a review of the published HIA report and interviews with five individuals, all of whom were members of the HIA steering group. The steering group included one current and two former members of staff from the Institute of Public Health but none of these individuals were interviewed.

Five semi-structured interviews were conducted over a one-month period from March to April 2006. Questions sent out in advance formed the basis for the interview. Interviewees included:

- a public health specialist from the regional Health Authority;

- the Director of Health Promotion from the local Health Authority;

- a senior engineer in traffic management from the City Council;

- the Assistant Programme Manager from a locally based EU-funded organization, with a remit to promote sustainable development in disadvantaged urban areas;

- a representative from the local community.

Profiling the HIA

Local-level concern that air-pollution levels were increasing in the locality led the Environmental Health Department of the city council to schedule an air quality and noise monitoring project for the area. At the same time a review of the Council's road safety plan in the local area was about to take place. The first phase of this, which fits into overall city development and transport plans, had been carried out in 2000 and included a number of initiatives to increase pedestrian and cyclist safety such as bollards and speed ramps, traffic islands, improved traffic signals, wider pavements and the introduction of cycle lanes. There had also been initiatives to improve public transport including a Quality Bus Corridor. As traffic congestion in the area was thought to be the main contributor to the perceived poor air quality, it was considered likely that any changes to traffic and transport recommended by this review would have an impact.

It was recognized that air quality was only one of the ways in which traffic and transport can impact on health. However, much of the evidence for this was anecdotal, particularly at local level. The HIA process was identified as a means of contributing to a wider understanding of these impacts, which in turn could influence future policy.

Initial discussions about undertaking an HIA began in 2003 and funding for the project was made available through the local Urban II office. This is a community initiative of the European Regional Development Fund (ERDF) for sustainable development in the troubled urban districts of the EU for the period 2000–2006 (ERDF, 2000). Due to the time scales involved in securing these funds, the review of the Road Safety Plan had already taken place. However, it was decided to proceed with the HIA as traffic and transport impacts on health had been identified as being of high importance to the local community. Also there was an interest in using the HIA as a learning project whereby the different organizations involved in the steering group could test the methodology and use it to inform future decisions.

The concept of HIA was understood as "a combination of procedures, methods and tools by which a policy, programme or project may be judged as to its potential effects on the health of a population, and the distribution of those effects within the population" (European Centre for Health Policy, 1999). The HIA was conducted at local level, in an urban district of a large city. The district has a population of approximately 20 000 and is recognized as an area of socioeconomic disadvantage. Its physical location, in a valley between two major arterial routes into the city centre, was thought to be a contributing factor to traffic congestion and the resulting stagnation of air.

An external consultant was engaged to guide the HIA process. The Merseyside Guidelines for Health Impact Assessment (Scott-Samuel, Birley & Ardern, 2001) were followed throughout the process. There was a general recognition of the broad determinants of health and this model was used to frame the HIA.

Most of the field work took place over a six-month period in 2004 and the report was launched in March 2005.

Aims and objectives of the HIA

According to the published report, the aim of the project was to conduct an HIA on transport initiatives in the local area and to use the findings and recommendations of the HIA to:

- influence the implementation of future transport policy including road safety initiatives in the local area;
- inform a review of the City Council's road safety plan;
- provide a health focus to an air quality and noise monitoring project being carried out at the same time by the City Council and funded by URBAN II;
- influence future health service development and delivery in the local area.

It was expected that the project would also:

- stimulate cooperation across the different sectors around initiatives which promote activities such as cycling and walking;
- engage the community to participate actively in decision-making by working in partnership with the statutory sector to influence planning and service development in the local area;
- promote understanding of the relationship between transport and health;
- develop learning around the practice of HIA.

The interviewees largely reiterated the objectives identified above although there were differences in the relative importance attributed to them. A relationship was noted between the objectives highlighted by a respondent and the remit of the organization that they were representing. For example, the city council representative was particularly interested in traffic management issues; future development of local services was seen as a priority for two respondents representing community interests.

Overall, respondents identified the main aim of the HIA to be assessment of the impact of traffic congestion, existing transport policy and/or traffic-calming measures on the health of the local community. There was a perception that traffic congestion was having a negative impact on health and it was felt that the HIA would help to clarify and quantify some of these issues.

Three respondents raised the issue of balancing different needs and expectation. From the perspective of the city council, there had to be a balance between this community and the larger city-wide setting:

> They were looking at the problem in isolation from the rest of the city but from our point we have to look at the whole city and specific measures to deal with this area will impact on other areas. It was difficult to explain this to community groups. They see their problem in isolation but they didn't see the regional or strategic view.

One local representative and a health professional noted differing needs even within the community itself. For example, traffic-policy benefits to pedestrians may impede motorists; restrictions introduced in one street may benefit that area at the expense of others.

The lack of one specific decision also meant that there were different expectations which had to be managed. For example, one of the community representatives spoke of her frustration at the HIA's focus on one specific issue:

> Initially I thought it was to look at the broad spectrum of health in the area, chronic disease, mental health etc. but because it coincided with work the Council wanted to do anyway I felt it steered away from this holistic picture and focused on the transport element.

The respondent who represented the main funding body was keen to ensure that the project fitted in with that organization's objectives:

> I wanted to ensure that the URBAN principles were applied to the process, that this resource was going to be useful to the

community, that it was real, not just broad recommendations that didn't really apply to anyone. Also making sure there was value for money for the community as it was funded by URBAN and that local knowledge was accessed and the community were adequately consulted.

From a community perspective, it was also felt that future health service development and delivery in the area could be influenced as the HIA would provide an overview of factors (e.g. smoking rates, physical activity, employment, education) influencing the health of local residents at both individual and community level, enabling a more targeted delivery of health services.

For three respondents (representing health authorities and the funding body) a major incentive for becoming involved with the HIA was to learn more about the methodology itself and to have the opportunity to apply this in a practical way. All of the respondents felt that involvement in the process would offer an opportunity to improve partnership working between the different sectors. This could benefit their work generally and/or improve local conditions.

Dimensions of effectiveness

General effectiveness

Two respondents felt that it was too soon to answer fully whether or not the HIA was effective and pointed out that a formal evaluation has not yet been carried out. However, in further discussions respondents made clear distinctions between the effectiveness of the HIA process, the implementation of recommendations and more long-term outcomes. This was summarized by one of the health representatives:

> If you look at the specific objectives, some were reached but others we don't know about yet. But it was key in raising awareness which is a very important first step. It also helped in learning about the HIA process.

The different levels at which effectiveness could be gauged were highlighted by three respondents, all of whom indicated that it was easier to cite specific examples of effectiveness at local level than more strategic changes. One of the community representatives said:

> At a local level there's now a group focusing on health in the area. It's great to have the report that can be used to influence policy locally, it can be used by politicians to try and get funding locally – it's a pressure document really.

Even where projects had been in place prior to the HIA, it was felt that their profile and uptake had benefited as a result.

It was more difficult to assess the HIA's impact on broader policy recommendations partly because of the policy-making process itself and where the HIA fitted into this, which again related back to its nature and timing. According to the council respondent, it is necessary to understand the way in which policy is formulated in order to make HIA more effective:

> A recommendation from a HIA, unless it was going to go through the city council structures, wasn't going to be implemented by the city council ... A report coming from an outside body wouldn't necessarily have the backing of the managerial staff or the elected members.

In addition, some interviewees expressed the view that the overall effectiveness of the project had been affected negatively because not all the key stakeholders had been invited to participate. For example, many issues were raised about the public bus service in the area, resulting in recommendations involving the service provider. However, this organization had not been identified and invited to participate from the outset.

Health, equity and community effectiveness

For the dimensions of effectiveness, there was a large degree of variation between the respondents regarding community and health effectiveness but more concurrence on equity. Analysis of the responses according to the organizations represented showed a clear distinction between responses from those representing the community and the city council. This may be related to position as those representing the community were based in the local area while the City Council representative was more central. Responses from the health representatives were somewhere between the two extremes. As noted in the sections above, it was easier to cite changes that had taken place at local level than changes to centrally driven policy.

From a community perspective there was a strong sense that the HIA was directly effective in terms of health, based largely on the findings of the community health profile and the literature review on traffic and health. It was felt that this information could be used to lobby for specific services in the future based on clearly documented health need. Representatives from the health authorities felt that health effectiveness was probably more opportunistic in that some recommendations bolstered projects which were likely to be implemented anyway. From the City Council's perspective it was felt that health was acknowledged but decisions were not altered because of the HIA.

Four of the respondents indicated general effectiveness regarding equity. It was felt that the process itself was equitable and that it highlighted equity issues within the community and between the community and elsewhere. For example, the area had one of the highest percentages of public bus usage in the city but was served by one of the oldest fleets. Within the community, the HIA highlighted issues of inequitable access to health and other local services which had been unknown to providers. However, one community respondent felt that this dimension of effectiveness was opportunistic. It is possible that such issues were already well known to the community but not to those outside the local area.

Both health and community representatives concurred that there was direct community effectiveness. This was the result of community involvement throughout the process: represented on the steering group and consulted through local groups. Also, community-based issues and decisions featured strongly in the recommendations. There were reservations about the management of expectations with different views about the extent to which this impacted on community effectiveness in the project. One respondent felt that while there were difficulties in terms of true engagement, there was still community effectiveness; another felt that this issue had not been addressed adequately and so the overall effectiveness of the community element of the HIA was reduced. According to one health representative:

> To truly engage with communities you need to have a way of handling and managing those priorities. So this was a weakness in our process, the closing of the loop was difficult; going back with findings was difficult because otherwise it's just consultation. If the community is going to be true partners then there needs to be more thought put into how we are going to prioritize and take all partners all the way in the analysis.

The importance of being clear about what the HIA could achieve and not raising false expectations when engaging with communities was elaborated further by one of the health respondents: "You need people within a management group to be reflective enough to differentiate between what was useful for the HIA and what was relevant for further work in the community."

All respondents highlighted organizational effectiveness as a positive outcome of the HIA process. The council respondent emphasized gaining insight into other organizations' work:

> Working with other agencies and learning what others are doing was informative and effective. I became aware of what Health Promotion was doing in schools and we were doing similar

work on road safety and walking or cycling to school. But if it was done together maybe we could have a more coordinated approach. So the process of the HIA rather than the outcome was effective in terms of having a better understanding of how different organizations operate.

In terms of the overall difference made by the HIA, one health representative talked about its contribution to future joint working:

A lot of the recommendations that came out for us would have been done anyway but that's not to say that the HIA wasn't worthwhile because for it to be reflected in a joint plan with ourselves and the council was really useful in terms of contributing to a solid partnership.

Factors influencing effectiveness

Process

Examination of the factors influencing effectiveness again raised the issue of which decision the HIA was attempting to influence, with different perspectives from different interviewees.

There were positive comments on the methodology and rigour of the HIA process and most respondents commented favourably on the appointment of an external HIA expert to guide the process. However, interviewees had different views on the scope of the HIA and responsibility for recommendations.

A screening tool was used but it appears that its purpose was to highlight elements for inclusion in the HIA rather than decide whether or not to proceed with the project. However, in discussing screening, respondents referred to the fact that a broader HIA for the area was considered but it was decided to limit the HIA to the area for which funds had already been secured and some degree of interest had been generated among the stakeholders.

A core working group, which included the two health professionals interviewed, gathered most of the data for presentation to the steering group. The latter had 20 members: representatives from the health services (4), city council (4), health research (3), academic or other research institutes (2), local community (4), an organization representing local community interests (2) and a planner from the Regional Transportation Office. All members of the steering group were involved in appraising the evidence, formulating recommendations and commenting on the final report. Priority recommendations were highlighted at an appraisal day at which participants were asked to identify five priority impacts, group them by themes and determine the level of evidence for this impact using predetermined guidelines.

Generally it was felt that there was a high degree of acceptance around the recommendations. Two respondents highlighted that some of the recommendations did not meet the original aims and objectives but only one saw this as problematic.

Overall it was felt that the community was involved from the beginning and included in representation on the steering group and wider consultation. Positive aspects of consultation were highlighted by four respondents and included using the services of an experienced qualitative researcher and facilitator, having pre-established links with community groups and sufficient time for the process.

In terms of paralleling different processes, one respondent felt that timelines were longer than anticipated for a number of reasons including administrative changes. Overall, there did not appear to be a sense of urgency about the process because the HIA was retrospective and not intended to influence a specific decision.

Input

A number of issues were raised concerning the driving forces for HIA. There was a keenness to test HIA methodology; use the process as a means of engaging, in some cases for the first time, with organizations in different sectors; and from the community perspective, a desire to have better access to health statistics for the community.

The main funders of the HIA were keen to get involved as it met their objectives of addressing community issues and using innovative methods for doing so. The driving forces from a health perspective appeared to be a combination of interest at policy level and personal motivation from the key drivers.

It took considerable time and effort to engage other stakeholders but it was felt that most decision-makers were represented throughout the process. However, while some organizations showed reluctance to become involved they were not totally opposed. It appeared that fear of the unknown was the major obstacle to some stakeholders becoming involved in the process. The issue of boundaries was raised by those who considered themselves to be drivers and those who were reluctant to engage with the process in its early stages.

There were mixed responses regarding future use of the report. One of the health respondents expressed the view that it had the potential to engage senior policy-makers about the health impacts of transport. The Council respondent pointed out that findings from areas within the remit of council activity (such as air quality and road accidents) had been found to be largely positive, therefore most of the recommendations were actually targeted at local areas rather than central implementation. However, the modification of local conditions would need to be seen in the context of the wider area. This representative also pointed out that the HIA was conducted on a council issue but the main drivers were from a health background, thus it would be seen ultimately as a health board initiative with findings which the Council could choose to dismiss.

Context

The contextual factors which influenced this HIA's ability to be influential or effective have been mentioned above.

In more general terms there was a mixed response to whether or not there is a public health culture. Health representatives felt that this was not really the case but others suggested that while the term public health may not be used or familiar to people, there was an understanding of the concept.

The general consensus was that HIA is not politically controversial but that may be because it has not been tested on particularly sensitive policies nor have there been situations where substantial negative impacts were identified as a result of the process. As it becomes used more widely it was thought that the likelihood will increase, particularly if HIA is established on a statutory basis.

In terms of facilitators and barriers, institutional capacity was seen as a positive in that some organizations were keen to get involved but it was felt that inclusion in job descriptions would have released more time to the process. Two respondents felt that legislative backing would have made it easier to engage with organizations and placed the onus on these organizations to comply with recommendations.

Conclusion

It was recognized that the retrospective nature of this HIA limited its scope to influence the decision-making process.

A formal evaluation has not yet been conducted and all respondents expressed the view that it was too soon to comment on the outcomes. There was general consensus that the process of engaging with HIA had been positive and had particularly highlighted the community's perspectives. It was also felt that this had facilitated working with other agencies and paved the way for future engagement.

Representatives from various health bodies were the main drivers behind this HIA and this continues to be the case in subsequent HIAs that have been conducted in Ireland. The newly formed Health Service Executive has identified HIA as a strategic priority in their 2005–2008 corporate plan (Health Service Executive, 2005), which is likely to give support to the future development of HIA.

REFERENCES

Department of Health and Children (2001). *Quality and fairness, a health system for you.* Dublin, Government of Ireland.

European Centre for Health Policy (1999). *Health impact assessment: main concepts and suggested approach. Gothenburg consensus paper.* Brussels, WHO Regional Office for Europe (http://www.euro.who.int/document/PAE/Gothenburgpaper.pdf, accessed 15 June 2006).

European Regional Development Fund (ERDF) (2000). *Urban II Initiative 2000–2006* [web site]. (http://ec.europa.eu/regional_policy/urban2/index_en.htm, accessed 15 June 2006).

Scott-Samuel A, Birley M, Ardern K (2001). *The Merseyside Guidelines for Health Impact Assessment. Second edition.* Liverpool, International Health Impact Assessment Consortium.

Moving towards the development of an HIA methodology: the effects of air pollution in Ticino, Switzerland

Konrade von Bremen

Introduction

Switzerland has 7.4 million inhabitants of whom 1.5 million are foreign nationals. The remaining 6 million speak three different languages: German (63%), French (20%) and Italian (6.5%), along with other languages. Canton Ticino's population of 350 000 is Italian-speaking but most of the inhabitants speak at least one other national language, if not two. The canton is divided geographically from the other regions by the Gotthard alpine pass, and its closest neighbour is the north Italian region of Lombardy. Canton Ticino's relative geographical isolation has produced a sense of autonomy among its inhabitants.

The Swiss Confederation is divided into 26 cantons that enjoy an important level of independence in most government affairs. Health care is one such area: Switzerland has 26 different and autonomous health-care laws and systems. Health impact assessment (HIA) is not a federal task and was, at the time of this evaluation (spring 2006), a cantonal affair.

Canton Ticino was selected for this case study because of its comprehensive approach to HIA through the cantonal Department of Health and Social Welfare, and for its high commitment to mainstreaming HIA in the government decision-making process. At the time the case was selected (January 2006) the

Office of Public Health had just received a report from the first comprehensive HIA. This undertook screening and scoping of health impacts relating to transport planning across the Alps through the region of Mendrisiotto, one of the best-known transport axes between northern and southern Europe. The choice of a transport-related HIA gave a new dimension to what had been purely health-related evaluations.

The context of this HIA can be explained by the complex political and administrative structure of Canton Ticino, and provides a strong example of basic democracy in a mature country. This basic democracy provided the basis for this HIA. The following section describes the profile of the HIA, provides insight into the process and gives an example of how political decisions may be made on behalf of a concerned population through an HIA approach.

The first aim of this project was to establish an appropriate methodology for HIA in the field of transport; precisely, one that allows exposure maps to be integrated with sociocultural parameters to relate air pollution exposure with health effects. An additional aim was to help to develop an HIA methodology suited, but not limited, to the transport sector. The methodology was followed as faithfully as possible to define parameters such as the costs and human resources necessary to implement HIA in the transport sector.

Transport across the Alps and associated problems

The Gotthard tunnel is one of the longest alpine tunnels, and one of the two preferred routes for public and private transport through the Alps; the other is the Brenner Tunnel in Austria. Most commercial transport is heavy vehicles transporting goods from the North Sea region to the Mediterranean countries (Filliger, Puybonnieux-Texier & Schneider, 1999). In the summer, tourism greatly increases the number of private vehicles on the motorway. This considerable transport load is not linked to the population of the Mendrisiotto region, the workforce and inhabitants of which very often commute between northern Italy and Switzerland. In the past, the commute was mainly from Italy to Switzerland; today the commute moves in both directions and adds to transport intensity in the region.

The level of fine powder air pollution is, therefore, well beyond the allowed limits and amongst the highest in Europe: 30 $\mu g/m^3$ compared to 20 $\mu g/m^3$ for the rest of Switzerland. In the Mendrisiotto region 70% of the population is exposed to these levels, compared to only 3% in the rest of the country (Jermini, 2005).

Using an epidemiological model it can be shown that the population is heavily exposed to air pollution, resulting in an 80% increase in pollution-related hospitalization and mortality.

Directives for the 2004–2007 legislative period adopted an innovative experimental approach which anticipated the integration of sustainability and health promotion; especially that related to equity, social integration and health effects of other policies. These directives reflect the sincere interest in HIA on the political level (Pesenti, 2005a; Pesenti, 2005b; Frei & Casabianca, 2006). This project is the first application of this strategy to use HIA as an instrument to increase internal consistency in public policy.

Collaboration and co-investment

The Office of Public Health within the Department of Health and Social Welfare is the institution with direct involvement in the HIA, with interest at three levels:

1 Operational: minimize negative health impacts and maximize positive impacts.
2 Strategic: link sustainability and health promotion through the HIA approach.
3 Methodological: develop methodological basis and competencies for further application and extended use.

As a political instrument in a direct democracy and in order to organize local and regional needs, Canton Ticino installed Regional Transport Commissions. These are composed of representatives from the county assembly of the surrounding villages and provide important input for transport planning and initiatives for better air and environmental quality. In this context, the President of Mendrisiotto's Transport Commission, a former railway worker, learned about HIA during a village event where an Office of Public Health representative convinced him that this approach could improve the quality of the regional transport strategy and help resolve some of the problems in the region. With the support of Mendrisiotto's entire transport commission he requested an HIA for one of the most polluted areas in Europe, as early as 2001. Following discussions at different levels the project was undertaken between 2002 and 2004. The feasibility report (screening and scoping of the transport plan) was delivered in 2005.

In order to perform any kind of HIA, a formal agreement between the Department of Territory and the Department of Health and Social Welfare was required. This uncustomary collaboration required a number of additional contacts and the creation of reference points. Political and personal changes in this new collaboration represented additional challenges for the project and prolonged the time frame in which it was performed. The Departments provided a joint mandate to undertake the HIA feasibility study in September 2002, and both contributed to the budget. The Office of Public Health provided HIA methodological support.

A local consultancy company with a proven and validated track record in environment assessment and urban planning was chosen to conduct the project. This company had no direct experience of addressing health questions but was ready to engage in the learning experience, convinced that the region needed a new approach for tackling pollution problems. Methodological hurdles were overcome with support from the Office of Public Health. The company reported that the experience was not easy but very positive, and confirmed their interest in undertaking other HIA projects. There was no discussion about whether projects in this field of public interest should be performed by a private company.

In January 2005 a cantonal resolution introduced HIA as an instrument for evaluating decisions in the health sector (Frei & Casabianca, 2006; Casabianca & Frei, 2004). An inter-departmental commission was put in place to implement the resolution, with the responsibility to propose a number of projects for an HIA evaluation. An innovative structure within the cantonal administration, the HIA Commission draws on the political will to establish HIA. It is composed of and coordinated by a staff member from Health Promotion in the Office of Public Health together with members from the Department of Territory. The Commission's task is to manage the evaluation process and evaluate whether the proposed solutions should be implemented. Normally, the Commission would use existing resources within the administration.

Aims of the HIA and dimensions of effectiveness

HIA is still in its infancy in Switzerland. The Department of Transport and the Department of Health and Social Welfare's joint effort to initiate this pilot project demonstrates their desire to perform pioneering work. They were well aware that all pilot projects require an extra time investment initially to establish processes and methodology.

The aim of the HIA was to develop a methodology that could be used for future HIAs – in this case, in the fields of transport and pollution. To understand the methodology used and the effectiveness of the HIA, interviews were conducted with four professionals who were directly involved.

The aims and results of the HIA were well illustrated by our four interviewees. The first was a public health specialist responsible for the development of HIA in Canton Ticino. He explained the complex local politics. His views on the project's aims focused on health policy and the opportunity to introduce HIA at a decision-making level. Despite the long evaluation period of nearly three years, the results met the level of expectations. Since the intention of the HIA was to develop an HIA methodology, rather than to influence a pending decision, clearly there could be no direct effectiveness. However, some of the interviewees felt there was general effectiveness in various areas. The public health specialist pointed out that effectiveness on health-related issues could not be evaluated in a screening and scoping exercise, because the HIA results were not implemented. Equity was strengthened with the project, as all levels of the population were directly involved and their concerns were considered equally. All affected regions were treated in an equal manner. The full effectiveness will only be appreciated when the HIA is implemented. Community effectiveness was confirmed by all three interviewees.

The second interviewee, a high-level public health specialist from the Office of Public Health, underlined the importance of this project for the canton and for the entire country. Equity effectiveness was respected but could not be fully shown in a scoping and screening exercise due to the missing implementation. Community effectiveness was achieved at a few levels. First, the community itself initiated the demand for an HIA, and this can be considered as 'effectiveness'. The responsibility of the project was almost entirely in the hands of community representatives, whether they were responsible for the transport commission or the local consultancy firm. At all phases, the community had full involvement in the project. The community representatives were only supported on methodological aspects from the public health specialist. The project initiator and promoter during the long period of the evaluation process was the community. All the interviewees stressed that this project showed high community effectiveness.

An unexpected form of effectiveness could be observed in this project: administrative effectiveness. The Department of Territory and the Department of Health and Social Welfare had few common tasks, and were not used to working together. This project obliged them to cooperate and together to define the objectives of the project. The hurdles in the project mainly involved new levels of cooperation and the political timetable, resulting in changes in people and their orientations. Even though it was not an intention at the beginning of the project, increased administrative effectiveness can be seen as one major success of the project.

The interviewee from the transport commission confirmed the above. He, a completely voluntary participant of the transport commission, convincingly showed that during a period of several years he attended project meetings at least every month, if not more. He confirmed the constant community involvement and therefore effectiveness of this HIA.

The fourth interviewee was responsible for the consultancy company that had performed the HIA. He described the project much more as a community member than as an external consultant. He and his company assumed the difficulties of a first pilot project in a new field. The initial methodological problems were readily solved in close collaboration with the Office of Public Health. The bigger hurdle was in the political arena, with changing responsibilities in different departments. It should be stressed that the project did not have to face clear opposition or major obstacles, although administrative pathways were sometimes long and burdensome. The interviewee concluded that it was a very positive experience and that he and his company would like to continue to work in the field of HIA, now that the basic methodological problems are solved. He strongly confirmed the community effectiveness as well as the administrative effectiveness at the end of the project. His involvement as a private company could suggest that this project was able to add another dimension of effectiveness that could be called 'economic or societal integration' (Gianmario Medici Studi Associati, 2005).

Process, input and context

The results of the report were presented to the Department of Territory and the Department of Health and Social Welfare. The department heads of the cantonal government were informed.

The specific characteristics of a direct democracy allow for direct community involvement at all times. In the context of Canton Ticino, individuals and their support activities have important roles in the decision-making process. This might be unique to Swiss democracy and most probably could not be translated into the context of another country.

Process

The current work started with preliminary discussions and a first draft offer in September 2001. In January 2002, the contract with the local consultancy firm was signed and the final report was delivered in September 2005 (Gianmario Medici Studi Associati, 2005). As HIA is not (in this context) an established evaluation tool, the first pilot study could be a screening and

Table CS17.1 *Social solidarity: actions and indicators*

	Actions foreseen by the Transport Commission	Possible indicators
Social solidarity	Reduce air particle emission rates by: • incentives to use public transport to reduce individual and private transport • promoting alternative technologies • promoting slow transport	Distribute emission charts Alternate people exposed on a regular basis
	Reduce noise emission rates by: • reducing speed • introducing speed limits (30 km/h) • various other actions	Distribute noise emission charts Alternate people exposed to excess noise levels
	Increase access to and improve public transport (e.g. intervals, connections)	Increase existing public transport Monitor users
	Promote 'Human-Powered Mobility'	Extend cycle paths Extend cycle-parking spaces
	Reduce accidents, especially involving infants Create 30 km/h zones Create pedestrian areas Build speed-limiting elements	Extend 30 km/h zones Monitor accidents

Source: Gianmario Medici (Studi Associati), 2005.

scoping exercise only. A full HIA had not been performed at the time of the assessment.

Wide determinants of health were taken into consideration including social solidarity and equity, or equal opportunities, to a large extent. Table CS17.1 shows the approaches taken according to these objectives of social solidarity.

Input

Inputs for the HIA in Ticino were provided by governmental initiative and support, and the community's request for an HIA. There were very low levels of opposition to this innovative initiative; none of the interviewees mentioned open opposition or clear opponents. It can be assumed that the public relevance of air pollution and the support from the Government and from the community gave a uniformly positive impulse for the project.

A large number of national and international associations and interest groups became involved with the project and actively supported the initiative, including the World Wide Fund For Nature (WWF), the Swiss Touring Club, the Rural Youth Association and the Industrial Association.

Context

The context of the HIA in Ticino shows a number of particularities when compared to other European countries or regions. The high level of political autonomy at cantonal level in the Swiss Federation is the background for the HIA's development. Switzerland has a strongly developed consensus culture at all public and even political levels. This explains the relatively smooth progress of the project in the political arena and at community level. Canton Ticino has a well-established public health culture and this provided the basis for the project.

Strategic environmental assessment (SEA) is another known assessment tool in Canton Ticino. The 1997 cantonal coordination law delegates responsibility for cantonal and regional transport plans: cantons set objectives for the infrastructure and evolution of transport. It is important to point out that an MP requested the integration of HIA within the environment assessment process in 1996 and 2001.

Conclusion

This chapter shows that HIA, even in methodological infancy, can be an important driving factor within its regional context. Today, HIA is on the political agenda in Canton Ticino because of this project and due to the strong community involvement. The HIA was conducted with the aim of stimulating decision-making and was not a reaction to a pending decision. This aim was achieved.

For the scoping and screening exercise, no direct health effectiveness could be shown. Equity effectiveness was not addressed explicitly, but was included in what is called social solidarity in Ticino. This aspect of equity was addressed strongly and as its determinants were included in the study, effectiveness has been achieved. Community effectiveness was achieved at a very high level and can be considered a major success. The marked and unexpected success of administrative effectiveness is due to the community and the fearless local consultancy company.

A health care professional with no direct involvement in the HIA concluded that it could be described as a very successful pilot study carried out in a real environment. It is thought to be worthwhile to implement the results of this first screening and scoping exercise as all the necessary elements are available for assisting the decision-makers.

REFERENCES

Casabianca A, Frei K (2004). *Switzerland: health impact assessment of Ticino's public policy.* Health Policy Monitor, Bertelsmann Stiftung, October (http://www.hpm.org/en/Surveys/USI/04/Health_Impact_Assessment_of_Ticino_s_public_policy.html, accessed 28 May 2007).

Filliger P, Puybonnieux-Texier V, Schneider J (1999). *PM10 Population exposure – technical report on air pollution.* Technical report, in Health costs due to road traffic-related air pollution – an impact assessment project of Austria, France and Switzerland. Bern, Federal Department of Environment, Transport, Energy and Communications, Bureau for Transport Studies EDMZ 801.630e.

Frei K, Casabianca A (2006). Health impact assessment: how the canton of Ticino makes health a common issue. *SPM,* 51:137–140.

Gianmario Medici (Studi Associati) (2005). *Piano dei trasporti del Mendrisiotto e Basso Ceresio (PTM). Valutazione dell'impatto sulla salute (VIS). Impostazione metodologica e proposte operative. [Transport plan for the Mendrisiotto region and the lower Ceresio (PTM). Evaluation of the impact on health (VIS). Design of the methodology and operational proposals].* Lugano, Studi Associati SA (http://www.ti.ch/DSS/dSP/SezS/pdf/VIS_PTM_Rapporto_finale.pdf, accessed 04 September 2007). Rapporto finale all'attenzione dell'ufficio di promozione e di valuazione sanitaria e dell'ufficio della protezione dell'aria [Final report to the health promoting section of the office of the air protection].

Gianmario Medici Studi Associati (2005). *Piano dei trasporti del Mendrisiotto e Basso Ceresio (PTM), valutazione dell'impatto sulla salute (VIS). Impostazione metodologica e proposte operative [Transport plan for the Mendrisiotto region and the lower Ceresio (PTM). Evaluation of the impact on health. Design of the methodology and operational proposals].* Rapporto finale all'attenzione dell'ufficio di promozione e di valuazione sanitaria e dell'ufficio della protezione dell'aria [Final report to the health promoting section of the office of the air protection]. Bellinzona: DSS Ufficio di promozione e valutazione sanitaria, DT Ufficio della protezione dell'aria (http://pre. ti.ch/DSS/DSP/SezS/pdf/VIS_PTM_Rapporto_finale.pdf, accessed 28 May 2007).

Jermini M (2005). Intervento di apertura del convegno [Opening discussion of the convention]. *Convegno scientifico, Salute e ambiente: l'impatto dello smog sulla salute della popolazione [Proceedings of the scientific convention, Health and environment: impact of smog on the health of the population].* Organizzato dal Gruppo Operativo Salute & Ambiente del Dipartimento della sanità e della socialità del Cantone Ticino [Organized by the Operative Group, Health and Environment of the Department of Health and Social Welfare of Canton Ticino], University of Lugano, 1 March 2005 (http://www.ti.ch/dss/temi/gos%2Da/convegni/ 1marzo2005/PDF/ Jermini010305.pdf, accessed 28 May 2007).

Pesenti P (2005a). Cosa può fare il Cantone? [What can the Canton do?] *Convegno scientifico, Salute e ambiente: l'impatto dello smog sulla salute della popolazione [Proceedings of the scientific convention, Health and environment: impact of smog on the health of the population].* Organizzato dal Gruppo Operativo Salute & Ambiente del Dipartimento della sanità e della socialità del Cantone Ticino [Organized by the Operative Group, Health and Environment of the Department of Health and Social Welfare of Canton Ticino], University of Lugano, 1 March 2005 (http://www.ti.ch/dss/temi/gos-a/convegni/1marzo2005/PDF/Pesenti010305.pdf, accessed 28 May 2007).

Pesenti P (2005b). La valutazione d'impatto sulla salute delle politiche pubbliche cantonali. Dall'obiettivo della sostenibilità all'impegno per il benessere dei cittadini [Evaluation of health impact of cantonal public policies. From the objective of sustainability to the engagement for the well-being of the citizens]. In: Dipartimento della sanità e della socialità CTS, ed. *Conferenza stampa del Dipartimento della sanità e della socialità del Cantone Ticino,* 17 January 2005 [press conference].

01 285786 030001 285786